DRUG OVERDOSES AND ALCOHOL WITHDRAWAL

PREVALENCE, TRENDS AND PREVENTION

SUBSTANCE ABUSE ASSESSMENT, INTERVENTIONS AND TREATMENT

Additional books in this series can be found on Nova's website under the Series tab.

Additional e-books in this series can be found on Nova's website under the e-book tab.

SUBSTANCE ABUSE ASSESSMENT, INTERVENTIONS AND TREATMENT

DRUG OVERDOSES AND ALCOHOL WITHDRAWAL

PREVALENCE, TRENDS AND PREVENTION

DAVID P. MORALES
EDITOR

nova
publishers
New York

NOTICE TO THE READER

Library of Congress Cataloging-in-Publication Data

Names: Morales, David P.
Title: Drug overdoses and alcohol withdrawal : prevalence, trends and
  prevention / editor, David P. Morales.
Description: Hauppauge, New York : Nova Science Publisher's, Inc., 2015. |
  Series: Substance abuse assessment, interventions and treatment | Includes
  index.
Identifiers: LCCN 2015036741 | ISBN 9781634838733 (hardcover)
Subjects: LCSH: Psychotropic drugs--Overdose. | Alcohol withdrawal syndrome.
  | Drug abuse--Social aspects--United States.
Classification: LCC RM315 .D793 2015 | DDC 615.7/88--dc23 LC record available at
http://lccn.loc.gov/2015036741

Published by Nova Science Publishers, Inc. † New York

CONTENTS

PREFACE

This book provides the latest research in substance abuse research. The first chapter evaluates psychotropic drug overdoses in forensic practices. Unintentional overdose deaths involving opioid pain relievers are discussed in the second chapter. In the next section, the prevalence, trends and management strategies for alcohol withdrawal are reviewed. The prolonged heavy drinking of alcohol (ethanol) often creates brain disorder alcoholism. In the third chapter, the authors explore alcohol withdrawal from the perspective of oxidative stress. Additionally, the authors discuss the epidemiology of alcohol withdrawal, the pathophysiology, and the diagnostic criteria for the various manifestations of alcohol withdrawal and management. Recent findings and new treatment options are reviewed as well.

Chapter 1 - Psychotropic drugs, including hypnotics, anxiolytics, antipsychotics, antidepressants, and anticonvulsants, are widely prescribed in routine medical practice. Overdose of psychotropic drugs is not uncommon in most advanced countries, and in these cases, multiple drug use is sometimes observed. Toxicological evaluation based on drug concentrations in blood or various samples is essential in forensic cases. Evaluation of poisoning due to multiple psychotropic drug ingestion constitutes a significant problem in the field of forensic toxicology because of the complexity of the pharmacological interactions among the various drugs, and the current lack of data and case reports for evaluation of multiple drug use. It has been reported that certain kinds of psychotropic drugs are especially toxic when combined with ethanol. Greater attention needs to be paid to the toxicity by combinations and interactions of multiple psychotropic drugs, including ethanol.

The cause of death in cases of psychotropic drug overdose may be mainly due to the depression of central nervous system (CNS) function. In most cases, non-specific findings, such as pulmonary edema, cerebral edema, and generalized organ congestion, can be obtained from macroscopic and microscopic examinations. The present paper discusses the pharmacology of psychotropic drug overdose and the importance of toxicological evaluation. The results of forensic toxicological evaluation may be able to contribute to the development of preventive measures for overdose.

Chapter 2 - Unintentional overdose deaths involving opioid pain relievers quadrupled from 1999 to 2007, surpassing those for heroin and cocaine. While there is a need for education on the prevention of opioid overdose, implementation of appropriate and potentially life-saving actions once an opioid overdose has occurred is necessary. Naloxone is a potent opioid antagonist indicated for the emergency treatment of known or suspected opioid overdose. It can be administered by several routes including intramuscular (IM), subcutaneous (SC), intravenous (IV), and intranasal (IN). Naloxone has been used for decades by healthcare workers for the treatment of known or suspected opioid overdoses. However, in recent years several states and large healthcare systems across the country have started distributing naloxone to individuals diagnosed with opioid use disorders and law enforcement agencies. This marks a new era in the treatment of opioid-related overdose.

Co-ingestants commonly occur with opioid overdose. Many opioids are commercially manufactured in combination with acetaminophen (APAP). Therefore, it is necessary to assess need of concomitant treatment of APAP toxicity in the setting of an acute overdose. N-acetylcysteine (NAC) is an antidote for APAP toxicity that prevents hepatic injury. Additionally, combining opioids with alcohol and/or sedative medication such as a benzodiazepine (BZD) increases the risk of respiratory depression and death. Flumazenil is a gamma-aminobutyric acid (GABA)$_A$ receptor antagonist used to treat BZD overdose that should be considered if concomitant BZD ingestion is suspected.

Antidotes for opioid and other common co-ingestants will be reviewed, including naloxone, NAC, and flumazenil. A detailed discussion of efficacy, pharmacology, pharmacokinetics, pharmacodynamics, adverse effects, and primary literature will be presented in this chapter.

Chapter 3 - The prolonged heavy drinking of alcohol (ethanol) often creates brain disorder alcoholism. Individuals with alcoholism experience a difficulty to control the amount of drinking in spite of adverse consequences. In particular, they encounter ethanol withdrawal (EW) syndromes upon a sudden cessation of drinking. The syndromes are largely hyperexcitatory (e.g., tremor, or seizure), due to an increase in excitatory neurotransmitters such as glutamate. Excessive glutamate overly activates its receptors, which in turn increases the entry of Ca^{2+} to the inside of cells and mitochondria. This exacerbates the generation of O_2 derived molecules, reactive oxygen species (ROS). While a moderate amount of ROS has been reported to be beneficial, the high amount of ROS overwhelms antioxidant enzymes and oxidizes cellular components, triggering cell damage, a phenomenon known as oxidative stress. Abundant evidence now indicates that EW stress damages the brain and other organs through mechanisms involving oxidative stress. During EW, ROS in concert with excitatory molecules provoke a wide range of oxidative stress including lipid peroxidation, protein oxidation, DNA oxidation, antioxidant suppression, and redox imbalance towards oxidation. These oxidative events may further interact with each other, amplifying neuronal damage. EW-induced oxidative stress warrants further research, which may ultimately help develop an adjunctive therapy for the successful detoxification of alcoholics who are not benefited by an existing therapy alone.

Chapter 4 - Alcohol Use Disorder and its myriad of complications are frequently encountered by Physicians each year. In the United States, it is estimated that approximately 8 million individuals suffer with Alcohol Use Disorder and approximately five hundred thousand will have symptoms of withdrawal, warranting some form of pharmacologic treatment each year. In individuals who are long-term alcohol consumers, reducing or stopping alcohol use suddenly leads to Alcohol Withdrawal Syndromes (AWS), a well-defined cluster of symptoms that range from mild tremors to withdrawal seizures and delirium tremens. In the United States, the estimated healthcare costs due to alcohol withdrawal, in 1998 was close to one hundred and eighty five billion dollars. Some of the costs of alcohol abuse such as domestic violence, child abuse, or loss of a future earnings and health were not even included in these estimates. Additionally, the morbidity and mortality associated with alcohol withdrawal makes it a topic of great importance. It is essential for physicians to be able to identify patients at risk of going into withdrawal and appropriately prevent, and manage all aspects of alcohol withdrawal so as to avoid the associated morbidity, mortality and costly hospital admissions.

This chapter will discuss the epidemiology of alcohol withdrawal, the pathophysiology, the diagnostic criteria for the various manifestations of alcohol withdrawal and the management. There are areas of controversy that exist in the clinical management of Alcohol withdrawal-where to treat and when and how to use medication-these will also be discussed. Recent findings and new treatment options will be reviewed.

Chapter 5 - Diseases and conditions in the elderly are generally characterized by numerous peculiarities. Diseases often tend to accumulate and potentiate each other. In geriatrics *multi-dimensionality* is typical. The elderly patient as a *bio-psycho-social unit* should be even more understood than those in the younger age group in both etiopathogenesis of diseases as well as in clinical practice. Psychological and social problems always appear simultaneously with somatic complaints, which also need to be handled with the same urgency. This applies for primary somatic diseases which are characteristic for advanced age (strokes, degenerative diseases, tumors, immobilisation). In a similar way this also applies for the so-called 'primary' mental disorders (dementia, depression, delirium) or so-called geriatric social syndromes (maladaptive geriatric syndrome; syndrome of mistreatment, neglect syndrome and elder abuse syndrome).

Majority of the clinical doctors consider multi-morbidity as an unpleasant phenomenon associated with the decrease in functional capacity, cognitive disorders, and moreover the risk of interactions between diseases themselves and their possible pharmacological therapy. In the elderly (especially late old age) multi-morbidity is the rule rather than the exception. Almost half of the people aged 65 to 69 years have two or more chronic diseases. The group of seniors with multi-morbidity has increased significantly especially in the last decade of life (22%). At the age of $\geq$ 85 y. there are more than 75% multi-morbid persons.

Pitfalls and negatives of multi-morbidity represent:

- Accelerated decline of the functional capacity
- The higher incidence of symptoms and subjective complaints
- The decline of quality of life
- Increased mortality
- Increased risk of hospitalization
- Increased risk of institutionalization (nursing or residential home, etc.)
- Rising health care costs

There is a lack of evidences for a specific treatment of multi-morbid seniors because they are usually excluded from major clinical trials (RCT = randomized clinical trials). The retrospective analysis of five general medical journals with the highest IF states that 284 of RCT from 1995 to 2010 65% of seniors were excluded for multi-morbidity. According to 11 Cochrane Review RCT assessment the presence of typical four chronic diseases (diabetes, heart failure, COPD, stroke) was less than half of the participants in these studies meeting the entry criteria either of the following chronic diagnoses. Multi-morbid seniors usually do not feature in the RCTs. Clinical guidelines generally do not count at all with multi-morbidity and often do not provide recommendations, which would take account of other simultaneously occurring comorbidities. Polypharmacy often justified and effective in the old age depends primarily on co-existing multi-morbidity. Although the individual diseases are quite correctly indicated and treated according to EBM (evidence-based medicine), quite often the possible impending pharmacological interactions recede into the background. Therefore it can be difficult to reveal it. Polypharmacy is also discussed in the situation when the patient is using only one not strictly necessary medicament. To some extent, this concept tends to lead to the noncoordination and the ineffectivity of therapeutic procedures. Polypharmacy may lead to an exponential increase of the risk of side effects and drug interactions (with 6 or more drugs is the risk particularly high according WHO).

The principles of geriatric prescription at a superficial glance may seem to give the impression that the prescription is similar to the one for younger individuals. The prescription for seniors requires understanding of: a clear indication of the drug; the knowledge of dosing; potential side reactions and drug interactions. In the geriatric prescription it is necessary to take into consideration the changes in cognitive function, decreased manual dexterity and vice versa the rise of the need of social support. The principles of prescription in the elderly comprise both the technical expertise of the prescription of drugs and the knowledge of bio-psycho-social factors enabling to meet all the individual needs of seniors.

The elderly are generally more vulnerable, the therapeutic range is narrowing, the compliance is decreasing, interindividual variability of the drug effect and the risk of drug interactions are increasing. In the elderly, there is a rise of gastric pH, on the other hand the stomach and intestinal motility as well as the blood flow to the gastrointestinal tract are decreasing. Despite all these changes the absorption of most drugs in the old age is not significantly affected.

In the elderly, about ½ patients aged 57-85 y. have ≥ 5 drugs. As the age is increasing, the number of drugs is increasing too. At about ½ of the cases wrong combination of drugs is prescribed (drug-drug) and about 1 in 20 has a high risk drugs combination.

The number of potential *drug interactions* grows exponentially with the number of drugs prescribed. The drug interaction may occur with some foodstuffs (absorption, metabolism). Potential side reactions are responsible for 1/5 of all hospitalizations of patients. It can be predicted that almost 1/3 and the mere reduction of the dose of medicament can be eliminated to 2/3 of them. Inappropriate medication by Beers criteria contributes only to 7% of hospitalizations.

Reduction of excessive polypharmacy is a benefit for the patient's health. It improves the treatment adherence and reduces the cost of medication. Scott directly states that no study has shown that the change (reduction) in polypharmacy decreased morbidity or mortality of seniors, but it led to a decline of potential side reactions (35%), costs decrease, and it also improved the compliance of the leftover medication. *The non-prescription of drugs should become a routine.*

The ideal situation of the geriatric prescription creates 1 prescribing doctor and 1 pharmacy. Each new physician increases the probability of potential side reactions by 29%. According to major studies e-prescribing can reduce inappropriate prescribing by 1-24%. Its effect on polypharmacy remains unclear.

Compliance decreases dramatically after ≥ 6 months of the drug usage. If the disease is symptomatic better adherence to the use of drugs occurs. The regular contact between the patient and the doctor is quite essential for improving and maintaining the adherence of an established therapy. Nothing can replace the 'face to face' visits at the doctor's office.

In: Drug Overdoses and Alcohol Withdrawal   ISBN: 978-1-63483-873-3
Editor: David P. Morales   © 2016 Nova Science Publishers, Inc.

Chapter 1

TOXICOLOGICAL EVALUATION OF PSYCHOTROPIC DRUG OVERDOSE IN FORENSIC PRACTICE

Hiroshi Kinoshita[1,], Naoko Tanaka[1], Ayaka Takakura[1], Mostofa Jamal[1], Asuka Ito[1], Shoji Kimura[1], Kunihiko Tsutsui[2], Shuji Matsubara[3] and Kiyoshi Ameno[1]*

[1]Department of Forensic Medicine
[2]Health Sciences, Faculty of Medicine, Kagawa University
[3]Community Health Care Education Support Center, and Postgraduate
Clinical Education Center, Kagawa University Hospital,
Miki, Kita, Kagawa, Japan

ABSTRACT

Psychotropic drugs, including hypnotics, anxiolytics, antipsychotics, antidepressants, and anticonvulsants, are widely prescribed in routine medical practice. Overdose of psychotropic drugs is not uncommon in most advanced countries, and in these cases, multiple drug use is

*All correspondence concerning this paper should be addressed to: Dr. H. Kinoshita, Department of Forensic Medicine, Faculty of Medicine, Kagawa University, 1750-1, Ikenobe, Miki, Kita, Kagawa, 761-0793, Japan. TEL: +81-87-891-2140 FAX: +81-87-891-2141. e-mail: kinochin@med.kagawa-u.ac.jp

sometimes observed. Toxicological evaluation based on drug concentrations in blood or various samples is essential in forensic cases. Evaluation of poisoning due to multiple psychotropic drug ingestion constitutes a significant problem in the field of forensic toxicology because of the complexity of the pharmacological interactions among the various drugs, and the current lack of data and case reports for evaluation of multiple drug use. It has been reported that certain kinds of psychotropic drugs are especially toxic when combined with ethanol. Greater attention needs to be paid to the toxicity by combinations and interactions of multiple psychotropic drugs, including ethanol.

The cause of death in cases of psychotropic drug overdose may be mainly due to the depression of central nervous system (CNS) function. In most cases, non-specific findings, such as pulmonary edema, cerebral edema, and generalized organ congestion, can be obtained from macroscopic and microscopic examinations. The present paper discusses the pharmacology of psychotropic drug overdose and the importance of toxicological evaluation. The results of forensic toxicological evaluation may be able to contribute to the development of preventive measures for overdose.

Keywords: Overdose, psychotropic drug, drug interaction, metabolism

INTRODUCTION

Drug overdose is a major public health problem [1, 2]. Poisoning is the second most common cause of unintentional death in the United States, and most of these deaths are due to overdose [3, 4]. There is a large amount of surveillance data from epidemiological studies [5-9]. It is known that the involvement of drugs differs significantly between countries, states and regions [1-9]. Clinical records [1, 10-13], autopsy records [14-17], and police statistics [18] show that overdose by psychotropic drugs is the most frequently observed cause of poisoning by pharmaceuticals in Japan. Overdose has a high incidence among users of sedatives-hypnotics, especially related to excessive dosage, barbiturate use, and multiple drug use [1, 14, 15, 17, 18].

Psychotropic drugs, including hypnotics (benzodiazepines, barbiturates, benzodiazepine-receptor agonists), anxiolytics (benzodiazepines), antipsychotics (phenothiazines, butyrophenones, heterocyclic compounds), antidepressants (cyclic antidepressants, selective serotonin reuptake inhibitors (SSRI), serotonin-noradrenaline reuptake inhibitors (SNRI)), and anticonvulsants (hydantoins, iminostilbenes, barbiturates, valproic acid) are widely prescribed in daily medical practice. Overdose by these drugs is a common problem in Japan [1, 10-18]. Forensic pathologists and toxicologists have a role to play in terms of medicolegal investigation. Detailed forensic patho-toxicological analysis in poisoning cases is useful, and data obtained by such studies is indispensable in enacting effective preventive measures. This paper provides an overview of autopsy, pharmacological, and toxicological findings in drug overdose, and may thereby contribute to the development of overdose prevention measures.

PHARMACOLOGY OF DRUG OVERDOSE

1) Hypnotics and Anxiolytics

Most hypnotics and anxiolytics are well and rapidly absorbed by the small intestine following oral ingestion [19, 20]. Most of these drugs are highly lipophilic. Therefore, clinical symptoms such as ataxia, incoordination, stupor or loss of consciousness are observed rapidly following ingestion [21]. These drugs act as central nervous system (CNS) depressants, due to the enhancement of the γ-aminobutyric acid (GABA)-mediated inhibitory neurotransmission [21]. Overdose can result in death from cardiorespiratory collapse by CNS and respiratory depression [19, 21].

2) Antipsychotics

Most antipsychotics are well absorbed by the gastrointestinal (GI) tract following oral ingestion [22]. As several of these drugs have anticholinergic properties, absorption by the intestine may be delayed by the decrease of GI motility, in case of massive ingestion [22, 23]. Overdose of antipsychotics causes a CNS depression, including impaired consciousness. It also causes prolongation of the QRS complex and QT interval in electrocardiogram (ECG). This may develop into fatal arrhythmia [22, 23].

3) Antidepressants

Most cyclic antidepressants are fairly well absorbed by the GI tract following oral administration [24]. Blood concentration of most cyclic antidepressants peaks within several hours of ingestion [24]. As several of these drugs have potent anticholinergic properties, absorption by the intestine may be delayed in an overdose by the decrease of GI motility [24, 25]. Most of these drugs are highly lipophilic and have a large distribution volume (V_d: 10-50L/kg), and are distributed to various organs [24]. Overdose of cyclic antidepressants causes cardiovascular toxicity, such as refractory hypotension, due to myocardial depression or prolongation of the QRS complex and QT interval in ECG [24, 26]. In the case of amoxapine overdose, incidence of seizures is significantly higher than that of other cyclic antidepressants [26-28]. Most SSRI overdoses cause CNS depression and cardiac toxicity, but these are usually not life-threatening [29]. However, since most SSRIs and their metabolites are substrates for, and potent inhibitors of, cytochrome P450 (CYP) enzymes, drug-drug interaction should be considered in cases of multiple drug overdose [24, 29-31].

4) Anticonvulsants

The mechanism of pharmacological action of anticonvulsants corresponds to one of the following mechanisms: sodium channel inhibition, calcium channel inhibition, inhibition of excitatory amines, or GABA agonism [32]. Overdose of carbamazepine causes a seizure and respiratory depression [33].

AUTOPSY FINDINGS IN DRUG OVERDOSE CASES

There may be no specific findings at autopsy in cases of psychotropic drug overdose. Since most psychotropic drugs cause no tissue damage in the gastrointestinal tract, even when ingested in large quantities, no evidence can be obtained by macroscopic or microscopic examination [34, 35]. Non-specific findings, such as edema and congestion of the lung, cerebral edema, and generalized organ congestion, have been observed in those cases [25, 34-42]. There may be remnants of undissolved tablets or granules formed by disintegrated tablets in the stomach [34, 38]. However, this is not always present in cases of drug overdose. Since there is no specific autopsy finding, it may not be possible to determine the cause of death by autopsy alone. We have to request detailed investigation through toxicological analysis [34].

TOXICOLOGICAL EXAMINATION

The forensic pathologist requests toxicological analysis for identification and quantification of drugs in the victim's blood, urine, stomach contents, or other specimens, collected at the time of autopsy [34, 35, 43, 44].

A conventional and commercial panel of immunoassays has been used as a screening test. Urine is usually collected for the sample of screening test, as it contains the ingested drug itself and its metabolites with fewer impurities [43]. Subsequent analysis for identification and quantification of drugs from blood, urine or other samples have been performed using instruments such as gas chromatography (GC), gas chromatography mass spectrometry (GC/MS), high performance liquid chromatography (HPLC) or liquid chromatography mass spectrometry (LC/MS) [43, 45, 46].

TOXICOLOGICAL EVALUATION

It is important to obtain as much information as possible regarding, for example, the past history of the deceased and ante-mortem signs or symptoms [34, 47]. Diagnosis of drug poisoning requires not only postmortem blood levels, but also the integration of other factors such as the clinical conditions and circumstances prior to death [47]. The forensic pathologist is concerned with the evaluation of the toxicity of drugs, and determines whether or not those drugs caused or contributed to death [34, 35]. The quantitative result of toxicological examination is important for proper diagnosis of poisoning. Numerous reference tables for fatal ranges of drug concentration have been reported, and these data can aid forensic diagnosis [34, 35, 43, 47]. However, since the postmortem blood concentration may be affected by various factors, as summarized in Table 1, these factors have to be taken into consideration for the evaluation of postmortem drug concentration [35, 43, 47, 48].

Table 1. Factors to be considered for evaluation of post mortem drug concentration

Sample and sampling time
Diffusion and redistribution
Degradation and formation
Drug interaction (drug-drug, drug-ethanol)
Metabolism

1) Samples and Sampling Time

The forensic pathologist usually collects blood as one of the autopsy samples for toxicological examination. The blood sample is preferably collected from the peripheral vein [34, 35]. The whole blood is usually used in a forensic analysis, as the separation of erythrocyte from serum is sometimes difficult because of the hemolysis by postmortem decomposition [35, 43, 47]. The composition of postmortem blood is also different to that of ante-mortem blood. It may depend on the postmortem interval. As the distribution of drugs is different to cellular components and serum, the concentration in whole blood and plasma differs with different drugs [35]. The drug levels determined by serum in a clinical setting do not always reflect the postmortem concentration in whole blood [35, 43, 47, 48].

2) Diffusion and Redistribution

The postmortem drug concentration in the intra-cardiac blood does not always reflect the concentration at the time of death [35, 43, 47, 48]. This may be due to two factors: diffusion and redistribution. There is a diffusion and redistribution of a drug from the stomach contents, organs, or aspirated vomitus in the trachea into surrounding tissue, including intra-cardiac blood [35, 43, 47-51]. This causes site-dependent difference of drug concentration in blood or tissue [52-55]. When we use a blood collected from the cardiac chamber as a sample for toxicological examination, we have to consider the effects of diffusion from stomach contents or vomitus, especially in cases of death by massive drug ingestion [49-55].

Postmortem redistribution is likely to occur in lipophilic basic drugs that have large V_d (> 3-4 L/kg) [47, 56]. This is due to the diffusion from the surrounding organs where the drug is highly accumulated. The liver, lung, and myocardium are major sources of redistribution in the postmortem period [51-56].

3) Degradation and Formation

Degradation of drugs could occur during the postmortem interval. This occurs as a result of bacterial invasion or continued metabolism by enzyme activity [47, 57]. The bacterial bioconversion of nitrobenzodiazepines such as flunitrazepam, nitrazepam, and clonazepam, has been studied [47, 57]. This causes formation of 7-amino-metabolite and disappearance or decrease of parent drugs in blood. In these cases, the presence of 7-amino-metabolite in blood would be an indicator of drug ingestion [37, 42, 58-63].

4) Drug Interaction

Most overdose cases involve more than one drug [14-18, 31, 36-41, 60-63]. In these cases, the drug-drug interaction would be taken into consideration. There are two types of drug interactions. One is pharmacokinetic interaction, which affects the drug concentration by altering the process of absorption, distribution, and metabolism [64]. As most psychotropic drugs are metabolized by CYP enzymes, competitive inhibition of the metabolic pathway by other drugs may occur [21, 23, 24, 29-31, 33, 61]. The other is pharmacodynamic interaction, which affects the response by changing its duration and severity [64]. The additive effects by two or more drugs in overdose potentiate the pharmacological action, and may cause a fatal outcome.

Since alcoholic beverages are popular in our daily life, there are many reports of drug interaction with ethanol [36, 42, 58, 60-63, 65-72]. Ethanol acts as a CNS depressant, and the action of psychotropic drugs is potentiated by co-ingestion with ethanol. These drugs are more dangerous in combination with alcohol than when taken alone [58, 72].

5) Metabolism

Most psychotropic drugs are metabolized in the liver or other organs. For example, imipramine is metabolized to desipramine, which has similar pharmacological activities to the parent drug [25]. We have to consider the concentration of active metabolite for the evaluation of toxicity [64].

CONCLUSION

In cases of drug overdose, collaboration between pathologist and toxicologist is essential for the detailed investigation necessary to determine of the cause of death. Autopsy findings and subsequent toxicological examination provide valuable information not only for determining cause of death, but also for taking effective preventive measures for overdose.

REFERENCES

[1]	Okumura Y, Tachimori H, Matsumoto T, Nishi D. (2015) Exposure to psychotropic medications prior to overdose: a case-control study. *Psychopharmacology* (Berl), 232, 3101-3109. doi: 10.1007/s00213-015-3952-8.

[2]	Paulozzi LJ, Annest JL. (2007) US data show sharply rising drug-induced death rates. *Inj Prev*, 13, 130-132. doi: 10.1136/ip.2006.014357.

[3]	Centers for Disease Control and Prevention (CDC). (2007) Increases in age-group-specific injury mortality – United States, 1999-2004. *MMWR Morb Mortal Wkly Rep*, 56, 1281-1284.

[4]	Centers for Disease Control and Prevention (CDC). (2011) Drug overdose death— Florida, 2003-2009. *MMWR Morb Mortal Wkly Rep*, 60, 869-872.

[5]	Centers for Disease Control and Prevention (CDC). (2004) Unintentional and undetermined poisoning deaths—11 states, 1990-2001. *MMWR Morb Mortal Wkly Rep*, 53, 233-238.

[6]	Centers for Disease Control and Prevention (CDC). (2005) Increase in poisoning deaths caused by non-illicit drugs—Utah, 1991-2003. *MMWR Morb Mortal Wkly Rep*, 54, 33-36.

[7]	Paulozzi LJ, Centers for Disease Control and Prevention (CDC). (2011) Drug induced death – United States, 2003-2007. *MMWR Morb Mortal Wkly Rep*, 60 Suppl, 60-61.

[8]	Paulozzi LJ. (2012) Prescription drug overdoses: A review. *J Safety Res*, 43, 283-289. doi: 10.1016/j.jsr.2012.08.009.

[9]	Jones CM, Mack KA, Paulozzi LJ. (2013) Pharmaceutical overdose deaths, United States, 2010. *JAMA*, 309, 657-659. doi:10.1001/jama. 2013.272.

[10]	Hirata K, Matsumoto Y, Tomioka J, Kurokawa A, Matsumoto M, Murata M. (1998) Acute drug poisoning at critical care departments in Japan. *Jpn J Hosp Pharm*, 24, 340-348.

[11]	Hirata K, Matsumoto Y, Matsumoto M, Murata M, Kurokawa A. (1999) Analysis of acute benzodiazepine poisoning cases in critical care departments and police agencies in Japan during 1996. *JAAM*, 10, 657-666.

[12] Asano H, Mori H, Yasuda C, Takeda A, Okada K, Mitsuda T, Yasuda T, Yamaguchi H. (2009) Analysis of cases of acute intoxication due to overdose in a suicide attempt using medicinal products. *J Jpn Soc Hosp Pharm*, 45, 201-204.

[13] Tashiro S, Sokabe S, Kuwahara K, Hashimoto T, Inoue D, Takata M, Hiraki Y, Yuki K, Manabe K. (2015) Examination of overdose patients that were admitted to the psychiatric ward after emergency transport. *J Jpn Soc Hosp Pharm*, 51, 452-455.

[14] Mizukami H, Mori S, Kato Y, Hamamatsu A, Tanifuji T, Dasai N, Hara S, Endo T, Misawa S. (2005) Possible influence of psychotropic drugs detected in blood when determining the cause of death in medicolegal autopsy cases in the Tokyo Medical Examiner's Office. *Nihon Hoigaku Zasshi*, 59, 149-159.

[15] Fukunaga T. (2012) Multiple prescription of drugs from the standpoint of Tokyo Medical Examiner's Office. *Japanese Journal of Psychiatric Treatment*, 27, 149-154.

[16] Nishimoto M, Nishiguchi M, Kitano K, Takeno Y, Suenaga S, Okudaira N, Nushida H, Nishio H. (2014) Forensic autopsy cases due to drugs and toxic substances in Hanshin area. *Acta Med Hyogo*, 39, 83-88.

[17] Fukunaga T, Tanifuji T, Suzuki H, Hikiji W. (2015) Psychoactive drugs and overdose deaths – report from Tokyo Medical Examiner's Office. *Japanese Journal of Psychiatric Treatment*, 30, 321-324.

[18] Tsunoda N. (1999) Drug and toxic poisoning in recent Japan. *Journal of Health Science*, 45, 356-366.

[19] Lee DC, Ferguson KL. (2011) Sedative-hypnotics. In: Nelson LS, et al. editors. *Goldfrank's toxicologic emergencies* (9th ed). pp. 1060-1071. New York, Chicago, McGraw-Hill.

[20] Kinoshita H, Tanaka N, Kuse A, Ohtsuki A, Nagasaki Y, Ueno Y, Jamal M, Tsutsui K, Kumihashi M, Ameno K. (2012) An autopsy case of triazolam overdose. *Rom J Leg Med*, 20, 297-298.

[21] Charney DS, Mihic SJ, Harris RA. (2006) Hypnotics and sedatives. In: Brunton LL, Lazo JS, Parker KL. editors. *Goodman & Gilman's the pharmacological basis of therapeutics* (11th ed). pp. 401-427. New York, Chicago, McGraw-Hill.

[22] Juurlink DN. (2011) Antipsychotics. In: Nelson LS, et al. editors. *Goldfrank's toxicologic emergencies* (9th ed). pp. 1003-1015. New York, Chicago, McGraw-Hill.

[23] Baldessarini RJ, Tarazi FI. (2006) Pharmacotherapy of psychosis and mania. In: Brunton LL, Lazo JS, Parker KL. editors. *Goodman &*

Gilman's the pharmacological basis of therapeutics (11th ed). pp.461-500. New York, Chicago, McGraw-Hill.

[24] Baldessarini RJ. (2006) Drug therapy of depression and anxiety disorders. In: Brunton LL, Lazo JS, Parker KL. editors. *Goodman & Gilman's the pharmacological basis of therapeutics* (11th ed). pp. 429-459. New York, Chicago, McGraw-Hill.

[25] Kinoshita H, Taniguchi T, Kubota A, Nishiguchi M, Ouchi H, Minami T, Ustumi T, Motomura H, Nagasaki Y, Ameno K, Hishida S. (2005) An autopsy case of imipramine poisoning. *Am J Forensic Med Pathol*, 26, 271-274.

[26] Liebelt EL. (2011) Cyclic antidepressants. In: Nelson LS, et al. editors. *Goldfrank's toxicologic emergencies* (9th ed). pp. 1049-1059. New York, Chicago, McGraw-Hill.

[27] Kulig K, Rumack BH, Sullivan JB, Brandt H. (1982) Amoxapine overdose coma and seizures without cardiotoxic effects. *JAMA*, 248, 1092-1094.

[28] Litovitz TL, Troutman WG. (1983) Amoxapine overdose seizures and fatalities. *JAMA*, 250, 1069-1071.

[29] Stork CM. (2011) Serotonin reuptake inhibitors and atypical antidepressants. In: Nelson LS, et al. editors. *Goldfrank's toxicologic emergencies* (9th ed). pp.1037-1048. New York, Chicago, McGraw-Hill.

[30] Goeringer KE, Raymon L, Christian GD, Logan BK. (2000) Postmortem forensic toxicology of selective serotonin reuptake inhibitors: a review of pharmacology and report of 168 cases. *J Forensic Sci*, 45, 633-648.

[31] Takahashi M, Kinoshita H, Kuse A, Morichika M, Nishiguchi M, Ouchi H, Minami T, Matsui K, Yamamura T, Motomura H, Ohtsu N, Yoshida S, Adachi N, Ueno Y, Hishida S, Nishio H. (2010) An autopsy case of poisoning with selective serotonin reuptake inhibitor, paroxetine. *Soud Lek*, 55, 2-4.

[32] Doyon S. (2011) Anticonvulsants. In: Nelson LS, et al. editors. *Goldfrank's toxicologic emergencies* (9th ed). pp. 698-710. New York, Chicago, McGraw-Hill.

[33] McNamara JO. (2006) Pharmacotherapy of the epilepsies. In: Brunton LL, Lazo JS, Parker KL. editors. *Goodman & Gilman's the pharmacological basis of therapeutics* (11th ed). pp. 501-525. New York, Chicago, McGraw-Hill.

[34] Knight B. (1996) *Forensic pathology*, (2nd ed), London, Arnold.

[35] Skopp G. (2010) Postmortem toxicology. *Forensic Sci Med Pathol*, 6, 314-325.

[36] Kinoshita H, Nishiguchi M, Kasuda S, Ouchi H, Minami T, Matsui K, Yamamura T, Motomura H, Otsu N, Yoshida S, Adachi N, Aoki Y, Nagasaki Y, Ameno K, Hishida S. (2008) An autopsy case of poisoning with ethanol and psychotropic drugs. *Soud Lek,* 53, 16-17.

[37] Kinoshita H, Nishiguchi M, Kasuda S, Takahashi M, Ouchi H, Minami T, Matsui K, Yamamura T, Motomura H, Otsu N, Yoshida S, Adachi N, Ohta T, Komeda M, Ameno K, Hishida S. (2008) Forensic toxicological implication of an autopsy case of mixed drug overdose involving clomipramine, chlorpromazine and flunitrazepam. *Soud Lek*, 53, 28-30.

[38] Kinoshita H, Morikawa K, Kuze A, Nagasaki Y, Takahashi M, Nishiguchi M, Nishio H, Ueno Y, Jamal M, Kubo Y, Tanaka N, Ameno K. (2010) An autopsy case of carbamazepine poisoning. *Soud Lek*, 55, 22-24.

[39] Tanaka N, Kinoshita H, Nishiguchi M, Jamal M, Kumihashi M, Takahashi M, Nishio H, Ameno K. (2011) An autopsy case of multiple psychotropic drug poisoning. *Soud Lek*, 56, 38-39.

[40] Kinoshita H, Tanaka N, Jamal M, Okuzono R, Kumihashi M, Ameno K. (2011) A fatal case due to multiple drug ingestion. *Current study of environmental and medical sciences*, 4, 3-5.

[41] Tanaka N, Kinoshita H, Kuse A, Takatsu M, Jamal M, Kumihashi M, Nagasaki Y, Asano M, Ueno Y, Ameno K. (2012) Forensic toxicological implications of pleural effusion; an autopsy case of drug overdose. *Soud Lek,* 57, 48-50.

[42] Tanaka N, Kinoshita H, Kumihashi M, Jamal M, Takakura A, Umemoto T, Tobiume T, Tsutsui K, Ameno K. (2014) Medicolegal implication of fatal poisoning by ethanol and psychotropic drug. *Current study of environmental and medical sciences*, 7, 3-5.

[43] Jones GR. (2008) Postmortem toxicology. In: Jickells S, Negrusz A. editors. *Clarke's analytical forensic toxicology.* pp. 191-217. London, Pharmaceutical Press.

[44] Suzuki O. (2002) How to handle biological specimens. In: Suzuki O, Watanabe K. editors. *Drugs and poisons in humans, a handbook of practical analysis.* pp. 1-7. Berlin, Heidelberg, Springer-Verlag.

[45] Suzuki O. (2002) Detection method. In: Suzuki O, Watanabe K. editors. *Drugs and poisons in humans, a handbook of practical analysis.* pp. 33-43. Berlin, Heidelberg, Springer-Verlag.

[46] Mofatt AC, Osselton MD, Widdop B, Jickells S, Negrusz A. (2008) Introduction to forensic toxicology. In: Jickells S, Negrusz A. editors.

Clarke's analytical forensic toxicology. pp. 1-11. London, Pharmaceutical Press.

[47] Kennedy MC. (2010) Post-mortem drug concentrations. *Internal Medicine Journal*, 40, 183-187.

[48] Moriya F. (2002) Pitfalls and cautions in analysis of drugs and poisons. In: Suzuki O, Watanabe K. editors. *Drugs and poisons in humans, a handbook of practical analysis*. pp. 17-24. Berlin, Heidelberg, Springer-Verlag.

[49] Pounder DJ, Yonemitsu K. (1991) Postmortem absorption of drugs and ethanol from aspirated vomitus –an experimental model. *Forensic Sci Int*, 51, 189-195.

[50] Pounder DJ, Fuke C, Cox DE, Smith D, Kuroda N. (1996) Postmortem diffusion of drugs from gastric residue: an experimental study. *Am J Forensic Med Pathol*, 17, 1-7.

[51] Moriya F, Hashimoto Y. (1999) Redistribution of basic drugs into cardiac blood from surroundings tissues during early-stages postmortem. *J Forensic Sci*, 44, 10-16.

[52] Jones GR, Pounder DJ. (1987) Site dependence of drug concentrations in postmortem blood – a case study. *J Anal Toxicol*, 11, 186-190.

[53] Pounder DJ, Jones GR. (1990) Post-mortem drug redistribution – a toxicological nightmare. *Forens Sci Int*, 45, 253-263.

[54] Pounder DJ, Adams E, Fuke C, Langford AM. (1996) Site to site variability of postmortem drug concentrations in liver and lung. *J Forensic Sci*, 41, 927-932.

[55] Pélissier-Alicot A-L, Gaulier J-M, Champsaur P, Marquet P. (2003) Mechanisms underlying postmortem redistribution of drugs: a review. *J Anal Toxicol*, 27, 533-544.

[56] Hilberg T, Ripel Å, Slørdal L, Bjørneboe A, Mørland J. (1999) The extent of postmortem drug redistribution in a rat model. *J Forensic Sci*, 44, 956-962.

[57] Robertosn MD, Drummer OH. (1995) Postmortem drug metabolism by bacteria. *J Forensic Sci*, 40, 382-386.

[58] Drummer OH, Syrjanen ML, Cordner SM. (1993) Death involving the benzodiazepine flunitrazepam. *Am J Forensic Med Pathol*, 14, 238-243.

[59] Moriya F, Hashimoto Y. (2003) Tissue distribution of nitrazepam and 7-aminonitrazepam in a case of nitrazepam intoxication. *Forensic Sci Int*, 131, 108-112.

[60] Kinoshita H, Nishiguchi M, Kubota A, Kasuda S, Ouchi H, Minami T, Matsui K, Yamamura T, Motomura H, Fujitomi Y, Ohta T, Tsuda T,

Hiromoto H, Hishida S. (2006) An autopsy case of fatal poisoning due to combined effects of ethanol and psychotropics. *Res Pract Forens Med*, 49, 39-43.

[61] Kinoshita H, Nishiguchi M, Kasuda S, Takahashi M, Ouchi H, Minami T, Matsui K, Ohtsu N, Yoshida S, Adachi N, Ameno K, Hishida S. (2008) An autopsy case of fatal poisoning due to combined effects of ethanol and psychotropics. *Forensic Sci Int*, 181, e7-8.

[62] Tanaka N, Kinoshita H, Jamal M, Ohkubo E, Kumihashi M, Ameno K. (2011) A case of drowning whilst under the influence of brotizolam, flunitrazepam and ethanol. *Soud Lek*, 56, 5-6.

[63] Kinoshita H, Tanaka N, Jamal M, Kumihashi M, Takakura A, Tobiume T, Tsutsui K, Ameno K. (2015) A fatal case of poisoning with ethanol and psychotropic drugs with putrefactive changes. *Soud Lek*, 60, 25-27.

[64] Drummer OH. (2008) Pharmacokinetics and metabolism. In: Jickells S, Negrusz A. editors. *Clarke's analytical forensic toxicology*. pp. 13-42. London, Pharmaceutical Press.

[65] Patel AR, Roy M, Wilson GM. (1972) self-poisoning and alcohol. *Lancet*, 300 (7787), 1099-1103.

[66] Stead AH, Moffat AC. (1983) Quantification of the interaction between barbiturates and alcohol and interpretation of fatal blood concentrations. *Human Toxicol*, 2, 5-14.

[67] Uemura K, Komura S. (1995) Death caused by triazolam and ethanol intoxication. *Am J Forensic Med Pathol*, 16, 66-68.

[68] Tanaka E, Misawa S. (1998) Pharamacokinetic interactions between acute alcohol ingestion and single doses of benzodiazepines, and tricyclic and tetracyclic antidepressants – an update. *J Clin Pharm Ther*, 23, 331-336.

[69] Tanaka E. (2002) Toxicological interactions between alcohol and benzodiazepines. *J Toxicol Clin Toxicol*, 40, 69-75.

[70] Tanaka E. (2003) Toxicological interactions involving psychiatric drugs and alcohol: an update. *J Clin Pharm Ther*, 28, 81-95.

[71] Kinoshita H, Nishiguchi M, Kubota A, Kasuda S, Takahashi M, Ouchi H, Minami T, Matsui K, Yamamura T, Motomura H, Ohtsu N, Yoshida S, Adachi N, Ohta T, Hiromoto H, Ameno K, Hishida S. (2008) A fatal poisoning case in a gastrectomy recipient due to the combined effects of psychotropic drugs and ethanol ingestion. *Japanese journal of foresic pathology*, 60, 25-27.

[72] Koski A, Ojanperä I, Vuori E. (2002) Alcohol and benzodiazepines in fatal poisonings. *Alcohol Clin Exp Res*, 26, 956-959.

In: Drug Overdoses and Alcohol Withdrawal   ISBN: 978-1-63483-873-3
Editor: David P. Morales   © 2016 Nova Science Publishers, Inc.

Chapter 2

OPIOID AND COMMON CO-INGESTANT ANTIDOTES

Emily E. Czeck[1]*, PharmD, BCPP
Andrea L. Quinn[2], BCPP, PharmD, BCPS
and Megan A. Rech[2,3], PharmD, BCPS
[1]Department of Pharmacy,
Battle Creek Veterans Affairs Medical Center;
[2]Department of Pharmacy,
[3]Department of Emergency Medicine,
Loyola University Medical Center

ABSTRACT

Unintentional overdose deaths involving opioid pain relievers quadrupled from 1999 to 2007, surpassing those for heroin and cocaine. While there is a need for education on the prevention of opioid overdose, implementation of appropriate and potentially life-saving actions once an opioid overdose has occurred is necessary. Naloxone is a potent opioid antagonist indicated for the emergency treatment of known or suspected opioid overdose. It can be administered by several routes including intramuscular (IM), subcutaneous (SC), intravenous (IV), and intranasal

---

* Corresponding author: Emily E. Czeck, PharmD, BCPP, Battle Creek Veterans Affairs Medical Center, Department of Pharmacy Services, 5500 Armstrong Road, Battle Creek, MI 49037, Phone: 330-207-7530, Emily.Czeck@gmail.com

(IN). Naloxone has been used for decades by healthcare workers for the treatment of known or suspected opioid overdoses. However, in recent years several states and large healthcare systems across the country have started distributing naloxone to individuals diagnosed with opioid use disorders and law enforcement agencies. This marks a new era in the treatment of opioid-related overdose.

Co-ingestants commonly occur with opioid overdose. Many opioids are commercially manufactured in combination with acetaminophen (APAP). Therefore, it is necessary to assess need of concomitant treatment of APAP toxicity in the setting of an acute overdose. N-acetylcysteine (NAC) is an antidote for APAP toxicity that prevents hepatic injury. Additionally, combining opioids with alcohol and/or sedative medication such as a benzodiazepine (BZD) increases the risk of respiratory depression and death. Flumazenil is a gamma-aminobutyric acid $(GABA)_A$ receptor antagonist used to treat BZD overdose that should be considered if concomitant BZD ingestion is suspected.

Antidotes for opioid and other common co-ingestants will be reviewed, including naloxone, NAC, and flumazenil. A detailed discussion of efficacy, pharmacology, pharmacokinetics, pharmaco-dynamics, adverse effects, and primary literature will be presented in this chapter.

OPIOID OVERDOSE AND TREATMENT

Introduction

All compounds related to opium are referred to as opioids. Opioids are available alone or in combination with other agents such as APAP. They have both analgesic and central nervous system (CNS) effects, with the potential to cause both euphoria and respiratory depression. Dependence and tolerance can develop to opioids. Dependence occurs due to changes in the locus ceruleus (LC). Norepinephrine is created in the LC and is attributed with stimulating wakefulness, breathing, blood pressure, and alertness. When opioids bind to mu receptors in the LC, norepinephrine release is suppressed. With repeated exposure to opioids, neurons in the LC modify their response and become hyperactive, offsetting the suppressive effects of opioids. If opioids are absent after this accommodation has been made, excessive amounts of norepinephrine are released resulting in withdrawal symptoms including anxiety, muscle cramps, diarrhea, and psychomotor agitation [1]. As a result of all these factors, there is a risk for overdosing on opioids. An opioid overdose is a medical emergency that requires prompt treatment including the opioid antagonist naloxone.

Prevalence

From 1999 to 2013 in the United States, drug poisoning deaths have more than doubled from 6.1 to 13.8 per 100,000 persons [2]. Whereas, drug poisoning deaths involving opioid analgesics have nearly quadrupled from 1.4 to 5.1 per 100,000. (Figure 1) In 2013, 43,982 drug overdose deaths were reported [3]. Prescription opioids account for 16,235 (37%) of these deaths, and 8,257 (19%) were from heroin. (Table 1) These statistics may underestimate the true burden of opioid overdose deaths as 22% of fatal poisoning records did not provide information on the involved drug [4]. The same year men were nearly four times more likely than women to die from a heroin-related drug-poisoning (6,525 versus 1,732 deaths, respectively), occurring most commonly between the ages of 25 and 44. In 2013, Non-Hispanic white persons aged 18-44 had the highest rate of drug-poisoning deaths involving heroin with 7 per 100,000. This is a drastic change from the year 2000 when non-Hispanic black persons aged 45-64 had the highest rate for drug-poisoning deaths involving heroin with 2.0 per 100,000 [4].

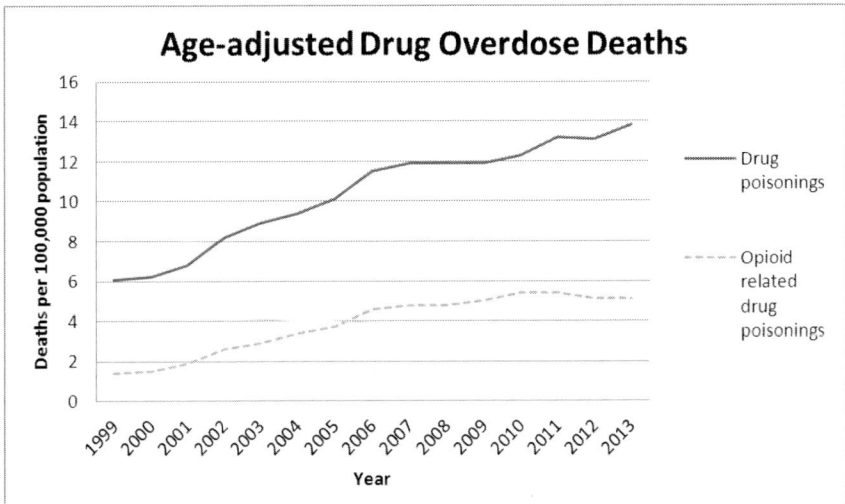

Figure 1. Age-adjusted Drug Overdose Deaths [5].

Table 1. Prescription Opioids

Prescription Opioids (listed alphabetically)		
Alfentanil	Hydromorphone	Oxycodone
Buprenorphine	Levorphanol	Oxymorphone
Butorphanol	Meperidine	Paregoric
Codeine	Methadone	Pentazocine
Dihydrocodeine	Morphine	Remifentanil
Fentanyl	Nalbuphine	Sufentanil
Hydrocodone	Opium	Tramadol

Common Co-Ingestants

In 2013, poison control centers in the United States reported 20,135 exposures to pure opioids resulting in 778 cases of major toxicity and 84 deaths. There were also 17,290 exposures to combinations of opioids with APAP, aspirin, or ibuprofen, with 308 cases of major toxicity and 52 deaths [6]. The use of opioids with BZDs has drastically increased. Thus, making knowledge of antidotes for opioids, APAP, and BZDs extremely beneficial [7].

Risk Factors

There are numerous factors associated with increased risk of opioid overdose, the first of which is increased availability of prescription and illicit opioids [8]. In the United States, there is a direct relationship between the number of opioid prescriptions, the dose prescribed, and overdoses [9]. Whereas, a decrease in the availability of heroin has been linked to a reduction in overdoses [8]. Another overdose risk factor is combining opioids with other substances. Both alcohol and BZDs are sedatives that effect GABA receptors in the CNS [10]. Respiration is mediated by GABA receptors and opioid receptors; therefore, the combination of opioids with alcohol or BZDs causes more potent respiratory depression than either alone [10]. Cocaine co-ingestion can also increase risk of opioid overdose. This is postulated to be due to impaired breathing associated with smoking "crack" or the onset of acute hypertension from the use of cocaine at the time of an opioid overdose [11].

Recent abstinence from opioid use including time spent in rehabilitation treatment programs or incarcerated also increases the risk of overdose [12].

Mechanism of Toxicity

The term toxidrome was first used in 1970 to describe a syndrome caused by dangerous levels of toxins [13]. The toxidrome for opioid overdose includes CNS depression with both respiratory and mental status changes, analgesia, miosis, orthostatic hypotension, nausea, and vomiting [14]. Opioids are the toxin responsible for this syndrome in an opioid overdose. They stimulate three primary opioid receptors: mu, kappa, and delta. These receptors are widely distributed throughout the body [15]. Activation of mu receptors results in analgesia, sedation, miosis, respiratory depression, cough suppression, euphoria, and decreased gastrointestinal motility. Two subtypes of mu receptors are well defined, mu_1 and mu_2. Respiratory depression has been consistently attributed to mu_2 receptors in the brain-stem [15, 16]. Through the activation of these receptors, opioids decrease ventilation by reducing medullary chemoreceptors sensitivity to hypercapnia [17]. Opioids also decrease respiratory response to hypoxia [18]. Hypercapnia and hypoxia stimulate respiration. Apnea is the result of decreasing the respiratory response to these circumstances. Constipation is the result of opioids binding to mu_2 receptors located in smooth muscle in the intestines [19].

Kappa receptor activation leads to some analgesic benefits, dysphoria, and possible hallucinations [16, 20]. Analgesia, cough suppression, and motor activity changes have all been attributed to delta receptors [21]. Opioid receptor-like receptors have also been identified as targets for endogenous opioids. The clinical role for this receptor is currently unclear [22]. Receptor activation varies depending on the specific opioid. However, all opioids have activity at mu receptors;, therefore, the ability to cause respiratory and mental status depression [23].

Diagnosis

Opioid poisoning is a clinical diagnosis based on recognizing characteristic signs and symptoms. The combination of respiratory rate less than 12 breaths per minute, miosis, and evidence of opioid use such as drug paraphernalia, needle marks, or bystander report has been found to be 92%

sensitive and 76% specific for diagnosing an opioid overdose [24]. Urine drug screens (UDS) are not routinely recommended for the diagnosis of an acute opioid overdose [25]. Naloxone administration should not be postponed in someone with respiratory depression while awaiting toxicology results as there is little variation in the treatment of an opioid overdose based on the specific agent. Also, standard UDS do not consistently detect semi-synthetic (i.e., hydrocodone, hydromorphone, oxycodone, oxymorphone) and synthetic opioids (i.e., fentanyl, meperidine, methadone),; therefore, adding minimal information to the diagnostic picture [26].

Treatment Strategies

In managing the overdose, the primary focus should be to address adequate oxygenation. Gastrointestinal decontamination with activated charcoal should be reserved for patients who present within one hour of ingestion or the treatment of potentially life-threatening co-ingestants [27]. Charcoal offers no benefit in the treatment of an opioid overdose beyond this time frame and can complicate treatment by obscuring visualization of the airway if intubation is necessary. For the reversal of an opioid overdose, naloxone is the standard pharmacologic treatment option. Naloxone was approved in 1971 by the Food and Drug Administration (FDA) as an antidote for opioid overdose [28]. It is an opioid antagonist at mu, kappa, and delta receptors. In the absence of opioids, usual doses of naloxone exhibit little to no pharmacologic activity. Tolerance has not been produced with repeated naloxone use nor has it been shown to create physical or psychological dependence.

Naloxone has poor oral bioavailability, but is well absorbed when injected IV, SC, or IM or when absorbed through mucosa after IN or endotracheal administration but not sublingual [29–34]. The onset of action varies depending on the formulation (Table 2). Naloxone is rapidly distributed in the body and readily crosses the placenta. Albumin is the main plasma protein bound by naloxone, but this binding is relatively weak. It is unknown whether naloxone is excreted into human milk. Naloxone is metabolized in the liver by glucuronide conjugation. The serum half-life in adults ranged from 30-81 minutes and in neonates from 3.1 ± 0.5 hours. Twenty-five to 40% of the drug is excreted as metabolites in urine within 6 hours of administration. Fifty percent is excreted in 24 hours, with 60-70% in 72 hours [35].

The dose of naloxone required depends on several factors including: amount of the opioid ingested or injected, relative receptor affinity for naloxone compared to the offending opioid, patient's weight, and presentation of the patient [36]. Recommended initial doses are shown in Table 2. Smaller doses (i.e., 0.2 mg) can be used to try to avoid withdrawal. However, it has been reported that twenty times the recommended dose of naloxone was required to counteract massive doses of opioids, even larger doses could be necessary if an overdose occurred in a body packer [37]. When the half-life of naloxone is shorter than the offending opioid, repeat administration or a naloxone infusion may be necessary. Continuous infusion should be considered if the patient is requiring multiple repeat administrations due to respiratory depression. To calculate the naloxone dose for continuous infusion, it is recommended to infuse two-thirds of the dose initially required for the observed patient response per hour [38].

**Table 2. Comparison of Routes of Administration
for Naloxone [30, 31, 35, 39]**

	IM	IN	SC	IV
Initial Adult Dose	Inject 0.4 mg in 1 mL	Spray 1 mg in 1 mL in each nostril	Administer 0.4 mg in 0.4 mL	Inject 0.4 mg in 1 mL to 2 mg in 5 mL
Repeat Doses if no Response	After 3-5 minutes	After 3-5 minutes	After 2-3 minutes	After 2-3 minutes
Onset	2-3 minutes	2-3 minutes	Longer than IV	Within 2 minutes
Time to "Response"	Mean 7.9 minutes	8-12.9 minutes	Mean 9.6 ± 4.58 minutes	Mean 9.3 ± 4.2 minutes, 8.1 minutes

Naloxone is relatively well-tolerated. Adverse effects are common, especially in individuals dependent on opioids. The most common adverse effects are related to opioid withdrawal and will occur within minutes of administration. These include nausea, vomiting, diarrhea, abdominal cramps, anxiety, piloerection, rhinorrhea, and yawning. Naloxone has been potentially linked to pulmonary edema. However, this relationship is unclear as pulmonary edema was reported in opioid overdoses before the development of naloxone [36].

To determine if a patient who has overdosed and stabilized after receiving naloxone should be discharged can be difficult. One study shows that if patients are independently mobile, have an oxygen saturation > 92% on room air, respiratory rate > 10 breaths per minute, normal temperature, heart rate > 50 beats per minute, and a Glasgow Coma Scale score of 15, they can be safely discharged one hour after naloxone administration when the opioid ingested is presumed to be heroin with a 99% sensitivity and 40% specificity [40]. If an individual who is walking and talking normally refuses to be observed for one hour after naloxone administration, the risk of developing potentially fatal respiratory or CNS depression was shown to be 0.17% [41]. If it is known or presumed that the opioid ingested was a substance other than heroin, it is recommended the individual be observed in the emergency department (ED) at least four to six hours after naloxone administration. The extended observation period is due to half-life differences between naloxone and opioids (Table 3) [42].

Table 3. Half-life Values for Selected Medications [35, 42, 43]

Medication	Half-life
Heroin	3.0 ± 1.3 minutes
Morphine	3-3.5 hours
Codeine	3 hours
Hydrocodone	2.5-4 hours
Oxycodone	2.5-3 hours
Hydromorphone	4 hours
Methadone	24 hours
Fentanyl	3-4 hours
Buprenorphine	3-5 hours
Naloxone	30-81 minutes

Administration by Laypersons

The majority of fatal overdoses occur in the company of others. However, , and that if medical help is often sought, it is often too late [14]. It is estimated that death from overdose occurs one to three hours after injection. Sixty-six percent of these deaths occurred in the home, and 85% occurred in the company of others. Despite observer presence, no ambulance was called on half these occasions. The death rate in heroin overdose managed at home is

10% [44]. One strategy to decrease the number of fatal opioid overdoses is distribution of naloxone for administration by laypersons if an overdose occurs.

Table 4. Advantages and Disadvantages of Layperson Administration of Naloxone by Route [39, 49–51]

	IM	IN	IM/SC Auto-injector
Advantages	Manufactured for this route Similar responder rates vs IV in prehospital setting	Reduce risk of needlestick injuries Reduce risk of blood-borne virus transmission Easy access to nares Reduces exposure to "triggers" for high risk individuals	Manufactured for this route Pocket-size; convenient; portable Retractable needle may reduce needlestick injuries Wide temperature storage range Easy to use for English-speaking non-hearing impaired individuals
Disadvantages	Risk of blood-borne virus transmission Risk of needlestick injuries Requires adequate dexterity for withdrawing dose from vial Requires adequate muscle mass for administration	Not manufactured for this route Nasal abnormalities and prior IN drug use may decrease effectiveness May have similar or lower responder rates and similar or slower onset than IM May be more likely to require supplemental dose (s)	May be difficult to use if voice instructions fail or if hearing loss present Small instructions on packaging that may be difficult to read if voice instructions fail Cost

Key organizations including the World Health Organization, United Nations Office on Drugs and Crime, American Medical Association, and American Public Health Association support the administration of naloxone by laypersons for the treatment of opioid overdoses [45–47]. In 2014, the Harm Reduction Coalition surveyed 136 organizations in 30 states that provided naloxone kits to laypersons. These organizations included public health departments, pharmacies, health care facilities, substance use treatment facilities, and community-based organizations, not including law enforcement organizations and emergency medical services.

They reported training 152,283 laypersons from 1996 through June 2014. One-hundred and nine of these programs provided data on 8,032 overdose reversals. Many organizations (50.7%) distribute only IM naloxone, 37.5% provided only IN naloxone, and both were available from 11.8% of the programs [48].

The cost-effectiveness of distributing naloxone to heroin users has been studied. Naloxone distribution to laypersons was found to be cost-saving by decreasing the number of overdoses and need for emergency services [52]. Using a "worst-case scenario" that included overdoses rarely being witnessed and naloxone rarely being used, minimally beneficial, and expensive, naloxone distribution was still concluded to be cost-effective with an incremental cost-effectiveness ratio of $14,000.

Overdose Prevention Strategies

Prevention is one key aspect to decreasing the number of opioid and other common co-ingestant overdoses. Strategies to reduce overdoses include education and family support groups [53]. The most effective method of decreasing mortality from overdose is opiate substitution programs. Methadone, an opioid agonist, and buprenorphine, a partial opioid agonist, are commonly used for such programs. Studies have demonstrated a reduction in incidence of fatal and non-fatal heroin overdoses with opioid maintenance programs [54, 55].

Methadone maintenance reduced heroin addicts' risk of death by 75% (risk ratio 0.25, 95% confidence interval 0.19 to 0.33) compared to no treatment [54]. However, access to these programs may be very limited, depending on geographic location [56].

Conclusion

As the number of opioid poisonings increase, education on treatment options and the antidote, naloxone, must also increase. This life-saving medication can be effectively administered by not only healthcare professionals but also by trained laypersons and can be administered via different routes to minimize risks associated with its use.

ACETAMINOPHEN OVERDOSE AND TREATMENT

Introduction

APAP is a common over-the-counter (OTC) analgesic and antipyretic that is frequently co-ingested with opioids due to multiple combination products available on the United States market (i.e., hydrocodone/APAP, oxycodone/APAP and codeine/APAP, among others). It is one of the most prolific OTC and prescription medications, and is available for adults and children in several dosage forms, including tablets, chewable tablets, suppositories, liquid, drops and IV preparations.

Prevalence

APAP is one of the most common agents implicated in overdose, both alone and in combination with other agents or other co-ingestants. Annually more than 30,000 patients are hospitalized for APAP toxicity, with liver injury occurring in 17% of adults with unintentional overdose [57]. Additionally, the proportions of patients with APAP hepatotoxicity caused by intentional versus unintentional overdose is almost equal, with the unintentional overdoses occurring more frequently from repeatedly exceeding the daily dose [58]. The Poison Control Center National Poison Data System reported 124,226 human exposures to APAP in 2013 [6]. APAP alone and in combination with other medications are listed as the 6th and 7th largest contributors to fatalities (all substances, including co-ingestants: n = 153 and n = 145, respectively; single substance ingestants: n = 44 and n = 58, respectively) [6]. This highlights the danger of overconsumption and co-ingestant with other sedatives and analgesics.

Recent steps have been made to combat this national health burden, including lowering the dose of APAP available in combination products (from 500 mg to 325 mg), reclassifying hydrocodone/APAP from a schedule III agent to a schedule II substance, thus limiting the number of prescribers and eliminating the ability to prescribe refills, and standardizing available pediatric formulations [59]. One multi-centered study of APAP-induced acute liver failure (ALF) showed that most overdoses (48%) in the United States are unintentional. Of the 662 patients meeting criteria for ALF, 275 (42%) were determined to result from APAP liver injury. Of these, 79% reported that they were taking the analgesic specifically for pain, and 38% were taking two different preparations of the drug simultaneously [58].

Mechanism of Toxicity

APAP causes predictable hepatotoxicity at supratherapeutic concentrations. The threshold for toxicity is 10-15 grams in adults and 150 mg/kg in children [60, 61]. At therapeutic doses (not exceeding 4 grams per day in adults), most of APAP is metabolized hepatically through a two-phase process via glucuronidation and sulfation and is subsequently excreted in the urine [61]. Approximately 5%-10% is metabolized by cytochrome P450 enzymes, primarily CYP2E1, to N-acetyl-p-benzoquinoneimine (NAPQI), a highly reactive toxic molecule that damages hepatocytes via covalent binding to proteins and nucleic acids, resulting in acute hepatic centrilobular necrosis [62–64]. NAPQI is detoxified when combined with glutathione to form water-soluble cysteine and mercapturic acid conjugates that are excreted in bile [65, 66]. At normal doses, there is enough glutathione to eliminate the toxic metabolite and prevent hepatotoxicity. Supratherapeutic APAP concentrations, either from a single exposure or chronic ingestion, can saturate sulfation, forcing more drug to be metabolized by glucuronidation and via CYP2E1, generating NAPQI in amounts that can deplete glutathione stores, resulting in liver injury [67, 68].

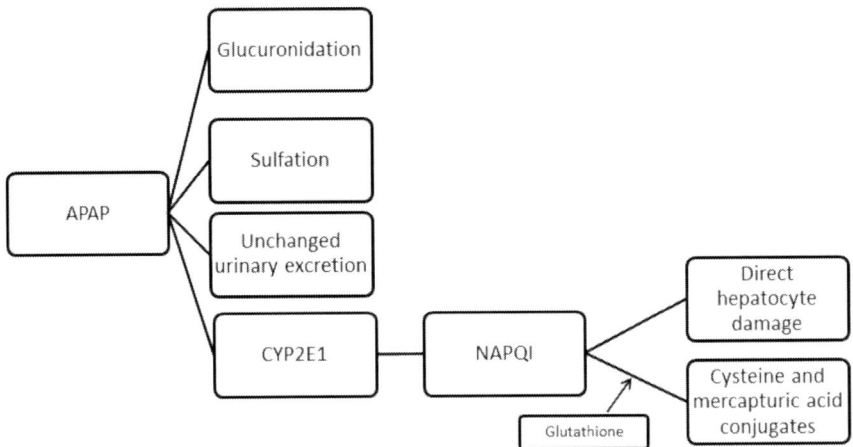

Figure 2. Metabolism of Acetaminophen.

Risk factors for toxicity include older age, late presentation, underlying hepatic disease, and genetic variation in cytochrome P450 morphology altering rate of APAP metabolism [69, 70]. Tobacco smoke, anticonvulsants, and isoniazid use have also been implicated as risk factors [60, 61, 71]. Acute alcohol intake may be protective as it is a competing substrate for CYP2E1, thus slowing the rate of NAPQI production [61, 72]. Chronic alcohol ingestion stimulates CYP2E1 activity and inhibits the rate of glutathione synthesis, resulting in increased toxicity [61, 70].

Presentation

There are four phases of toxicity associated with APAP overdose, depending on the time from ingestion [61, 72]. In early overdose (phase 1, within 24 hours), patients typically present with non-specific symptoms of nausea, vomiting, malaise, and abdominal pain [73]. In phase 2 (24 to 72 hours), symptoms may improve or even disappear. Hepatic injury may ensue 2 to 3 days after ingestion with right upper quadrant pain and tenderness. Serum transaminase, aspartate aminotransferase (AST), and alanine aminotransferase (ALT) levels may increase as early as 12 hours, but typically 24-36 hours after ingestion [73, 74]. Phase 3 occurs 3 to 5 days post-ingestion, liver injury peaks, leading to coagulopathy, encephalopathy, and jaundice. Hepatocellular injury and death most commonly occur during phase 3 [73, 75]. Phase 4 occurs from day 4 and thereafter, and includes resolution of liver damage and symptoms thereof [72]. A study in the United Kingdom reported fewer than 10% of patients with APAP overdose would develop severe liver damage, and only 1% to 2% would develop ALF [76].

Diagnosis

Serum concentrations of APAP are readily available at most institutions and should be drawn if there is clinical suspicion of overdose. Levels should be drawn at 4 hours post-acute ingestion. Levels before four hours should not be relied upon to exclude toxicity [77]. The Rumack-Mathews nomogram, which plots APAP concentrations against time from acute ingestion, is a useful tool to determine risk of hepatotoxicity [78]. Patients with a four hour concentration greater than 200 mcg/mL or above a line drawn from the four hour mark to 24 hours corresponding to the half-life are at high risk of hepatic injury and should be treated with the antidote NAC. A parallel line at 150 mg/mL at four hours demonstrates *possible* hepatoxicity. This threshold is most commonly used in the United States to determine if treatment is necessary [78, 79]. Of note, this nomogram only extends up to 24 hours post-ingestion and should not be used for presentations beyond this point. A recent retrospective case series of acute APAP ingestion found that 62% of patients had APAP levels drawn before the four hours post-ingestion [80]. These levels were associated with an increased likelihood of not obtaining optimally timed concentrations, therefore, not appropriately applying the Rumack-Mathews nomogram to determine if treatment is necessary, resulting in unnecessary use of NAC. Therefore, for acute ingestion, levels should not be drawn prior to four hours post-ingestion.

Treatment Strategies

Prompt recognition and treatment is imperative to prevent liver injury and ultimately death. After acute ingestion, activated charcoal can be considered to reduce the absorption of APAP, though there is limited data to support its use, and it may interfere with the adsorption of antidote therapy [81, 82]. It should ideally be administered within one hour of ingestion [60, 72]. Gastric lavage and syrup of ipecac should generally be avoided [81].

NAC is a widely-accepted antidote that prevents hepatic injury primarily by restoring hepatic glutathione [83]. NAC greatly reduces the incidence of hepatotoxicity and progression to fulminant liver failure when used within 8-10 hours of acute ingestion [79, 84]. The largest study to date studied oral NAC in 2540 patients and found that hepatotoxicity developed in 6.1% of patients at probable risk when NAC was started within 10 hours of APAP ingestion [79]. NAC should also be considered in patients presenting after this time if demonstrating symptoms of ALF. One small retrospective study of patients treated from 10 – 36 hours after ingestion found that NAC was associated with a 21% reduction in mortality [85].

NAC is available via IV or oral administration for APAP overdose. The IV dosing regimen consists of a bolus of 150 mg/kg followed by 50 mg/kg over 4 hours and then 100 mg/kg over 16 hours [79]. If the patient is able to take oral medications, NAC is available in a solution that is dosed at 140 mg/kg, followed by 70 mg/kg orally every 4 hours for 17 doses [79]. The latter is preferable as this route is generally more benign; however, it may be difficult to tolerate due to its pungent odor and taste. Most commonly, side effects include nausea and vomiting, and if a dose is vomited, it must be repeated. (61,67) It may be diluted with juice or water to improve potability. In addition to gastrointestinal symptoms, IV administration may result in rash, pruritus, bronchospasm, rhinorrhea, and infusion reactions, including fevers, chills, angioedema, hypotension, and anaphylaxis [61, 86]. No studies have directly compared IV to oral administration of NAC [67, 81].

Though not often necessary due to the efficacy of NAC, use of extracorporeal treatments may be considered as well. APAP is moderately dialyzable, with one study demonstrating that 11% of a 650 mg dose was removed with 3 hours of hemodialysis [87]. The Extracorporeal Treatments in Poisoning (EXTRIP) workgroup suggests that extracorporeal treatments should be implemented in patients with excessively large overdoses who display features of mitochondrial dysfunction, including early development of altered mental status and severe metabolic acidosis prior to hepatic failure onset [88].

Though data is limited and of low methodologic quality, the EXTRIP group recommends hemodialysis for patients with: APAP concentration >1000 mg/L if NAC is not administered, signs of mitochondrial dysfunction and an APAP concentration >700 mg/L if NAC is not administered, and signs of mitochondrial dysfunction and an APAP concentration >900 mg/L if NAC is administered.

Liver transplantation may be considered in cases of APAP-induced fulminant hepatic failure (FHF) Transfer to the intensive care unit of a medical center with a liver transplantation program should be arranged if patients are at risk of FHF [89, 90]. Liver transplantation improves long-term survival. A large retrospective study of FHF patients demonstrated a 5 year survival rate of 67% [91]. Most patients were comatose, on hemodialysis, and ICU-bound before transplantation.

Conclusion

APAP is commonly co-ingested with opioids due to availability in combination products and OTC preparations. Prompt recognition and treatment is necessary to prevent progression to ALF. NAC is the mainstay of therapy.

BENZODIAZEPINE OVERDOSE AND TREATMENT

Introduction

BZDs are a class of psychoactive medications that are often referred to as 'tranquilizers', 'benzos', 'nerve pills', or 'downers' [92]. The most commonly prescribed BZDs include alprazolam, lorazepam, clonazepam, diazepam, and temazepam, and according to the Drug Enforcement Agency (DEA), these same agents are also the most likely to be used for illicit purposes [92]. Although the exact reason for the frequency of nonmedical use is unknown, it may be hypothesized that the spike correlates with prescription frequency. Other BZD agents include midazolam, oxazepam, and the older agents, chlordiazepoxide and triazolam. BZDs are commonly prescribed for anxiety disorders, alcohol withdrawal, skeletal muscle relaxation, rescue medication for seizure disorders, and preoperative and pre-procedural sedation and amnesia. Specific indications vary between agents according to pharmaco-kinetic differences between agents [92, 93].

Most BZDs are available as oral and injectable agents with diazepam also available as a rectal gel. Illicit BZD users have been reported to 'snort' BZDs either as single agents or to combat untoward effects with use of IN illicit agents like methamphetamine or heroin [94].

These drugs carry a higher risk of patient hospitalization, impaired cognition and motor function, increased fall risk in elderly patients, and increased risk of physical and psychological dependence [93]. Agents with a rapid onset are more likely to produce the euphoric effects potentiating the risk of abuse. BZDs are often used in combination with opioids or with other illicit agents to enhance euphoria or counteract the untoward effect of concomitant agents [92].

Prevalence

It is estimated that 5.2% of adults in the United States aged 18 to 80 years have filled at least one prescription for a BZD and use increases with age. Younger patients (aged 18 to 35 years) report the lowest prescription use at 2.6% while older patients (aged 65 to 80 years) report the highest prescription use at 8.7% of patients [93]. In 2011 alone, 126 million prescriptions for BZDs were dispensed with alprazolam accounting for 49 million, which is increased from the estimated 44 million alprazolam prescriptions dispensed in 2008 [92, 95].

ED visits associated with nonmedical use of BZDs continue to increase. According to the Drug Abuse Warning Network (DAWN), BZD associated visits increased by 141% from 1995 to 2005 [96]. Hospitalizations in the United States for poisoning by prescription sedatives, tranquilizers and opioids increased 65% from 1999-2006, and BZD poisoning accounted for the largest increase in the number of hospitalized cases. Furthermore, those patients were most likely to present to a rural or urban nonteaching hospital and were more likely to be women aged 34 years or older. ED visits for nonmedical use of BZDs increased by an additional 89% from 2004 to 2008 with a shift towards the younger population ages 21-29 years. Nonmedical BZD use is often accompanied with other co-ingestants as BZDs were reported to be involved in 26% of opioid related visits and alcohol was involved in up to 25% of BZD related ED visits [95]. According to DAWN, on an average day in 2011, there were 2,317 drug related visits to the ED by individuals aged 18 to 25 years with 1,340 of these visits involving illegal drugs, pharmaceutical abuse or misuse, or alcohol in combination with other drugs. Of the visits, 228 involved BZDs, either in combination with other agents or as single entities [97].

There were 38,329 drug overdose deaths reported in the United States in 2010 alone, and of these deaths, 57.7% involved pharmaceutical agents with BZDs accounting for 29.4% of these drugs either as single entities or in combination [98]. The 2010 National Survey on Drug Use and Health estimated 186,000 new abusers of BZDs with data correlating to increased opioid co-ingestion in an effort to enhance the opioid 'high' [99]. BZD use was involved in 31% of opioid related deaths in 2011 [2].

The 2013 Annual Report of the American Association of Poison Control Centers' National Poison Data System (NPDS) denote the class of sedatives/hypnotics/antipsychotics as the fifth most frequent drug class involved in all human exposures for which a call or internet inquiry was made at 5.9% (n=2,188,013) [6]. The total number of substances associated with the 1218 fatalities reported during this time frame was 2822 and sedatives/hypnotics/antipsychotics were reported as the leading substances (12.86%). However, during this time frame there were only 538 events (3.5%) reported as single drug exposure with sedative/hypnotics/antipsychotics. This information suggests that BZD overdose as a single agent is relatively rare.

The frequency of use and abuse is not surprising. The 2002 to 2009 report from the National Ambulatory Medical Center Survey (NAMCS) from 2002 to 2009 reportshows that of the 3.1 billion primary care visits included in the analysis, 12.1% involved a prescription for an opioid or BZD, with BZD prescription rates increasing by 12.5% annually and BZD co-prescription rates by 12% per year [100].

Despite BZD classification as a schedule IV controlled substance, there are mechanisms in which BZD may be obtained by individuals for illicit use. Unethical health care providers can divert medications or sell fraudulent prescriptions. Patients may 'doctor shop' and visit numerous physicians in order to get several prescriptions. Individuals may try to have fraudulent prescriptions filled or alter legal prescriptions to increase the quantity or number of refills. Moreover, BZD can be stolen from individuals who have legitimate prescriptions which stresses the importance of keeping medications is in a safe and secure place [92, 101].

Mechanism of Toxicity

BZDs act on the post-synaptic $GABA_A$ receptor. This receptor consists of 5 glycoprotein subunits: 2 α subunits, 2 β subunits and 1 γ subunit. The BZD receptor is located on the α subunit and is classified as a BZD_1 or BZD_2 receptor based on clinical effect [102]. The BZD_1 receptor contains the α_1 isoform, which is present in sixty percent of $GABA_A$ receptors and concentrated in the cerebellum, cortex and thalamus. The BZD_2 receptor contains the α_2 isoform and is primarily located in the limbic system, motor neurons and the dorsal horn of the spinal cord. Sedation, anterograde amnesia, and some of diazepam's anticonvulsant effects are affiliated with the BZD_1 receptor, while the anxiolytic effects of these agents appear to be mitigated through the BZD_2 receptor [102].

BZDs elicit their CNS depressant action via nonselective binding to the BZD_1 and BZD_2 receptors on the post-synaptic $GABA_A$ receptor. This binding enhances GABA's inhibitory effect on neuronal excitability by increasing membrane permeability to chloride ions which results in hyperpolarization of the neuron and increased stabilization. BZD agonism by binding to BZD_1 receptor results in increased sedation while binding to the BZD_2 receptor results in cognition, memory, and psychomotor impairment. However, not all BZDs interact with the same BZD receptor or with the same affinity to a specific receptor. This nonselective variability in binding to the BZD receptors is responsible for both the therapeutic and adverse effects [102, 103].

Ensuant to this mechanism of action, CNS effects are the most commonly reported adverse reactions. Sedation, dizziness, drowsiness, impaired cognition, slurred speech, memory loss, and impaired psychomotor skills, which can lead to an increased risk of falls, can occur. These effects can also appear over time as BZDs are slowly eliminated from the body and repeated doses can lead to accumulation in fatty tissues [102]. Euphoria has been reported and is most often associated with rapid onset BZD, which leads to the increased risk of abuse [92, 102]. These adverse effects can be intensified when BZD are combined with other agents, like opioids or alcohol, and respiratory depression increases in a dose dependent manner when BZD are taken in conjunction with opioids. Patients with chronic obstructive pulmonary disease carry an increased risk of respiratory depression with BZD use [102]. Therapeutic levels and toxic levels have been reported for some, but not all of the BZDs (Table 5).

Table 5. Therapeutic and Toxic Levels of Select BZDs [104, 105]

BZD	Therapeutic range (ng/mL)	Toxic range (ng/mL)
Alprazolam	10-50	32-162
Chlordiazepoxide	700-1000	>5000
Clonazepam	15-60	>80
Diazepam	100-1000	>5000
Lorazepam	50-240	Not established
Oxazepam	0.2-104	Not established

Acute toxicity is a result of the BZD mechanism of action and the specific BZD pharmacologic properties (Table 6) [102].

Presentation

The clinical manifestation of suspected BZD toxicity is dependent on the route of exposure and the presence of co-ingestants. Presentation varies as the pharmacologic characteristics and BZD receptor binding affinity of BZDs differ between agents, but the toxidrome generally manifests as augmentation of the CNS depressant effect with approximately normal vital signs [106].

Symptoms following acute ingestion of single-entity BZD are often mild in nature and generally reversible. Severe toxicity with BZD as a single agent and fatality are rare [106].

Table 6. Pharmacokinetic Comparison of Select BZDs

Agent	Comparative oral dose (mg)	Protein binding	Volume of distribution (Vd) L/kg	Metabolism	Onset	Time to peak concentration (hours)	Half-life (hours)
Alprazolam	0.5	80%	0.84-1.2	n/a	Intermediate	IR: 1-2 XR: 9	6-27
Diazepam	5	PO: 98%	PO: 0.8-1	Hepatic	Rapid	0.25-2.5	44-48
Lorazepam	1	85-93%	1.3	n/a	Intermediate	~2	~12
Temazepam	30	96	1.4	n/a	Intermediate – Slow	1.2-1.6	3.5-18
Clonazepam	0.25	85	41.5-64.5	n/a	Intermediate	1-4	17-60

PO = Oral IR = Immediate Release XR = Extended Release.

However, the effects of the BZD in conjunction with co-ingestants like alcohol or other sedative-hypnotic agents can be enhanced and may result in severe CNS depression, as previously mentioned [102, 107]. Other clinical manifestations that can be seen include dysarthria and ataxia. Although coma is rare, it can occur in elderly patients [107].

Symptoms following IN or IV BZD use mimic those seen after oral ingestion. Pharmacokinetic parameters vary after oral, IV and IN use. Intranasal BZD use has been shown to have a rapid onset and bioavailability ranges from 38% to 98% [108]. Intentional or inadvertent intra-arterial BZD administration may lead to phlebitis or severe vascular impairment. Depending on the agent, symptoms may be mild and resolve or severe and require surgical intervention [109, 110].

Table 7. Common symptomology following toxic BZD ingestion

Organ System	General presentation	Symptoms correlated with severe toxicity
Cardiovascular	Bradycardia, sinus tachycardia	Hypotension, Cardiac arrest
CNS	Amnesia, ataxia, CNS depression, drowsiness, hallucinations lethargy, sedation, slurred speech	Coma, hypothermia
Gastrointestinal	Abdominal pain, nausea, vomiting	
Ocular	Nystagmus	

Diagnosis

The diagnosis of BZD toxicity is made upon physical examination, patient history, laboratory assessment and clinical suspension. Urine, saliva, blood, sweat, and nails are some of the biological specimens that may be used in drug screens [111]. Point-of-care or on-site qualitative urine immunoassays to determine the presence of a specific drug or metabolite are utilized most frequently in health care institutions due to the quick turnaround time. Unfortunately, false positives and false negatives have been associated with qualitative assessments. Oxaprozin, a non-steroidal anti-inflammatory agent, and sertraline, a selective serotonin reuptake inhibitor antidepressant agent, are two agents that can cause false positive results for BZD [111]. Quantitative assays via gas chromatography or mass spectrometry to determine the specific amount of the ingestant are also available. These assays are not practical in an acute setting due to the prolonged turnaround time and are not widely used. Assay availability is dependent on institution preference.

Treatment Strategies

The treatment mainstay for BZD toxicity is resuscitation and supportive care, including maintaining adequate oxygenation and blood pressure and preventing aspiration [107]. Clinical controversy surrounds the use of gastric decontamination. Syrup of ipecac induces vomiting, but due to the risk of aspiration pneumonia, it is no longer recommended. Gastric lavage may be considered; however, airway protection is critical. There is lack of data supporting improved clinical outcomes and use carries morbidity and mortality risks including gastrointestinal tract perforation and aspiration [107]. Although, many drugs may be absorbed by activated charcoal, efficacy of this agent is time dependent, repeat doses may lead to bowel obstruction, and there is lack of evidence showing beneficial clinical outcome [107, 112].

Flumazenil is a specific BZD antagonist that was FDA approved in 1991. It acts as a competitive antagonist at the $GABA_A$ BZD receptor and may be considered in the treatment of BZD overdose or for the reversal of BZD sedative effects in conscious sedation. Re-sedation has been reported in patients after initial response [106]. Flumazenil does not antagonize CNS effects of other GABA agonists including barbiturates or ethanol as these agents bind to different sites on the receptor [102].

Flumazenil carries a Black Box warning regarding seizure development. Patients taking BZDs long-term or who are suspected of having a tricyclic antidepressant overdose are at an increased risk of seizure development following flumazenil administration due to precipitation of withdrawal symptoms and removal of the BZD seizure protective effects [106, 113]. Furthermore, use may unmask cardiac arrhythmias once the BZD protective effects are removed [106]. Although successful use has been reported with diagnostic differentiation of mixed-agent toxins and coma of unknown etiology, manufacturer drug information cautions against flumazenil use as a diagnostic agent as the toxic effects of the co-ingestant (s) may emerge once the BZD effects are reversed [114]. Secondary to the inherent risks, flumazenil is rarely indicated in the acutely poisoned patient unless it is known with certainty that a BZD was the only agent ingested and that the patient has no history of seizures.

BZD toxicity is rapidly reversed following flumazenil administration. Adult dosing for suspected BZD overdose is 0.2 mg IV push over 30 seconds to 1 minute via a freely running IV into a large vein. (106) Product information suggests that a 0.3 mg dose can be given if the desired level of consciousness is not obtained 30 seconds after the initial dose. Should re-sedation occur, especially in the setting of conscious sedation reversal, repeat flumazenil doses may be given every 20 minutes. The incidence of re-sedation development is greatest with midazolam doses of 10 mg or more or use of a long acting BZD due to the agent's prolonged half-life. Hypoventilation associated with BZD ingestion is not consistently reversed following flumazenil administration and others causes should be considered. No more than 3 mg of flumazenil should be administered in one hour [106]. Adverse effects per manufacturer data Include vomiting, palpitations, ataxias, dizziness and vertigo [114]. Flumazenil is only available via generic pharmaceutical manufacturers as 0.1 mg/ml in 5 mL or 10 mL vials. Cost ranges from $8.15 (5 mL) to $15.60 (10 mL), but with the increasing amount of drug shortages, manufacturer consistency and drug supply cannot be guaranteed.

Conclusion

BZDs are one of the most frequently prescribed pharmacological classes of medications, yet toxicity from use as a single agent is rare. BZD use is often combined with alcohol or opioid analgesics, and practitioners must remember to assess patients for possible co-ingestants. The mainstay of treatment in an overdose situation is supportive care. Flumazenil specifically antagonizes BZD effects; however, caution should be advised against routine administration. Although use may be considered in patients who present with BZD toxicity as a single agent, use should be avoided in patients with a history of seizure disorders, long term BZD use, or unknown co-ingestant status as the risks of use outweigh the potential benefit.

CONCLUSION

With the continued increase in the number of opioid overdose deaths, healthcare professionals should improve their knowledge of treatment strategies including supportive care and antidote administration. Since opioids are often ingested with APAP and BZDs, it is prudent for these professionals to also understand the available antidotes for these agents. Naloxone, an opioid antagonist, NAC, a modified amino acid, and flumazenil, a $GABA_A$ antagonist are all effective antidotes for treating toxicity for their respected target agents. Their doses, routes of administration, time to effect, and half-life values vary and are all facts that should be considered in the management of an overdose. These treatments options also have adverse effects that providers should anticipate and be prepared to manage. Mastery of this information improves patient care in the event of an overdose.

CONFLICTS OF INTEREST

Financial support was not received for chapter preparation. None of the authors have conflicts of interest to disclose

REFERENCES

[1]   Kosten TR, George TP. The neurobiology of opioid dependence: Implications for treatment. Sci Pract Perspect [Internet]. 2002 [cited 2015 Jul 30]; Available from: http://archives.drugabuse.gov/pdf/ Perspectives/vol1no1/03Perspectives-Neurobio.pdf
[2]   Chen L, Hedegaard H, Warner M. Drug-poisoning deaths involving opioid analgesics: United States, 1999-2011 [Internet]. Centers for Disease Control and Prevention (CDC) Drug U.S. *Department of Health and Human Services NCHS Data Brief*, No 166. 2014 [cited 2015 Jul 28]. Available from: http://www.cdc.gov/nchs/data/databriefs/db166.htm
[3]   Chen L, Hedegaard H, Warner M. QuickStats: Rates of Deaths from Drug Poisoning and Drug Poisoning Involving Opioid Analgesics — United States, 1999–2013. MMWR Morb Mortal Wkly Rep. 64 (01):32.
[4]   Hedegaard H, Chen LH, Warner M. Drug-poisoning deaths involving heroin: United States, 2000-2013 [Internet]. US Department of Health and Human Services, Centers for Disease Control and Prevention, *National Center for Health Statistics*; 2015 [cited 2015 Jul 27]. Available from: http://198.246.124.29/nchs/data/databriefs/db190.pdf
[5]   Data Brief 190: Drug-poisoning deaths involving heroin: United States, 2000-2013 [Internet]. Centers for Disease Control and Prevention (CDC)

National Center for Health Statistics. [cited 2015 Jul 30]. Available from: http://www.cdc.gov/nchs/data/databriefs/db190_table.pdf

[6]   Mowry JB, Spyker DA, Cantilena LR, McMillan N, Ford M. 2013 Annual Report of the American Association of Poison Control Centers' National Poison Data System (NPDS): 31st Annual Report. *Clin. Toxicol.* 2014 Dec;52 (10):1032–283.

[7]   Paulozzi L, Weisler R, Patkar A. A national epidemic of unintentional prescription opioid overdose deaths: how physicians can help control it. *J. Clin. Pychiatry.* 2011;72 (5):589–92.

[8]   Prescription painkiller overdoses in the US | VitalSigns | CDC [Internet]. [cited 2015 Jul 28]. Available from: http://www.cdc.gov/vitalsigns/ painkilleroverdoses/index.html

[9]   Bohnert AB, Valenstein M, Bair MJ, et al. Association between opioid prescribing patterns and opioid overdose-related deaths. *JAMA.* 2011 Apr 6;305 (13):1315–21.

[10] Dietze P, Jolley D, Fry C, Bammer G, Moore D. When is a little knowledge dangerous? Circumstances of recent heroin overdose and links to knowledge of overdose risk factors. *Drug Alcohol Depend.* 2006 Oct 1;84 (3):223–30.

[11] Warner-Smith M, Darke S, Lynskey M, Hall W. Heroin overdose: causes and consequences. *Addiction.* 2001;96 (8):1113–25.

[12] World Health Organization. Prevention of acute drug-related mortality in prison populations during the immediate post-release period. Copenhagen, Denmark: World Health Organization, Regional Office for Europe; 2010. 25 p.

[13] Mofenson HC, Greensher J. The nontoxic ingestion. *Pediatr Clin. North Am.* 1970 Aug;17 (3):583–90.

[14] Sporer KA. Acute heroin overdose. *Ann. Intern. Med.* 1999;130 (7):584–90.

[15] Stein C. The control of pain in peripheral tissue by opioids. *N. Engl. J. Med.* 1995 Jun 22;332 (25):1685–90.

[16] Sheffler D, Roth B. Salvinorin A: the "magic mint" hallucinogen finds a molecular target in the kappa opioid receptor. *Trends Pharmacol. Sci.* 24 (3):107–9.

[17] Weil J, McCullough R, Kline J, Sodal I. Diminished ventilatory response to hypoxia and hypercapnia after morphine in normal man. *N. Engl. J. Med.* 292:1103–6.

[18] Lalley PM. Opioidergic and dopaminergic modulation of respiration. *Respir. Physiol. Neurobiol.* 2008 Dec;164 (1-2):160–7.

[19] Holzer P. Opioids and opioid receptors in the enteric nervous system: from a problem in opioid analgesia to a possible new prokinetic therapy in humans. *Neurosci. Lett.* 361 (1-3):192–5.

[20] Millan M, Czonkowski A, Lipkowski A, Herz A. Kappa-opioid receptor-mediated antinociception in the rat. II. Supraspinal in addition to spinal sites of action. *J. Pharmacol. Exp. Ther.* 1989;251 (1):342–50.

[21] Henriksen G, Willoch F. Imaging of opioid receptors in the central nervous system. *Brain.* 2007 Nov 29;131 (5):1171–96.

[22] Courteix C, Coudoré-Civiale M-A, Privat A-M, Pélissier T, Eschalier A, Fialip J. Evidence for an exclusive antinociceptive effect of nociceptin/orphanin FQ, an endogenous ligand for the ORL1 receptor, in two animal models of neuropathic pain: *Pain.* 2004 Jul;110 (1):236–45.

[23] Chahl L. Opioids - mechanisms of action. Aust Prescr Indep Rev [Internet]. 1996 [cited 2015 Aug 3];19. Available from: http://www.australianprescriber.com/magazine/19/3/63/5

[24] Hoffman J, Schriger D, Luo J. The empiric use of naloxone in patients with altered mental status: a reappraisal. *Ann. Emerg. Med.* 1991 Mar;20 (3):246–52.

[25] Boyer EW, Shannon MW. Which drug tests in medical emergencies? *Clin. Chem.* 2003 Mar;49 (3):353–4.

[26] Shaw L. The clinical toxicological laboratory: contemporary practice of poisoning evaluation. Washington, DC: AACC Press; 2001.

[27] Clarke S, Dargan P, Jones A. Naloxone in opioid poisoning: walking the tightrope. *Emerg. Med. J. EMJ.* 2005 Sep;22 (9):612–6.

[28] Yap D. Old drug, new life: naloxone access expands to community pharmacies [Internet]. American Pharmacists Association. 2015 [cited 2015 Aug 3]. Available from: http://www.pharmacist.com/old-drug-new-life-naloxone-access-expands-community-pharmacies

[29] Dowling J, Isbister GK, Kirkpatrick CMJ, Naidoo D, Graudins A. Population pharmacokinetics of intravenous, intramuscular, and intranasal naloxone in human volunteers. *Ther Drug Monit.* 2008 Aug;30 (4):490–6.

[30] Robertson TM, Hendey GW, Stroh G, Shalit M. Intranasal naloxone is a viable alternative to intravenous naloxone for prehospital narcotic overdose. *Prehosp. Emerg. Care.* 2009 Jan;13 (4):512–5.

[31] Wanger K, Brough L, Macmillan I, Goulding J, MacPhail I, Christenson JM. Intravenous vs subcutaneous naloxone for out-of-hospital management of presumed opioid overdose. *Acad. Emerg. Med.* 1998;5 (4):293–9.

[32] Merlin MA, Saybolt M, Kapitanyan R, Alter SM, Jeges J, Liu J, et al. Intranasal naloxone delivery is an alternative to intravenous naloxone for opioid overdoses. *Am. J. Emerg. Med.* 2010 Mar;28 (3):296–303.

[33] Sabzghabaee AM, Eizadi-Mood N, Yaraghi A, Zandifar S. Naloxone therapy in opioid overdose patients: intranasal or intravenous? A randomized clinical trial. *Arch. Med. Sci. AMS.* 2014 May 12;10 (2):309–14.

[34] Pond SM, Tozer TN. First-pass elimination. Basic concepts and clinical consequences. *Clin. Pharmacokinet.* 1984 Feb;9 (1):1–25.

[35] Naloxone hydrochloride injection, USP, opioid antagonist [Package insert]. Lake Forest, IL: Hospira, Inc; 2008.

[36] Boyer EW. Management of opioid analgesic overdose. *N. Engl. J. Med.* 2012 Jul 12;367 (2):146–55.

[37] Schneir AB, Vadeboncoeur TF, Offerman SR, Barry JD, Ly BT, Williams SR, et al. Massive OxyContin ingestion refractory to naloxone therapy. *Ann. Emerg. Med.* 2002 Oct;40 (4):425–8.

[38] Goldfrank L, Weisman RS, Errick JK, Lo MW. A dosing nomogram for continuous infusion intravenous naloxone. *Ann. Emerg. Med.* 1986 May;15 (5):566–70.

[39] Kerr D, Kelly A-M, Dietze P, Jolley D, Barger B. Randomized controlled trial comparing the effectiveness and safety of intranasal and intramuscular naloxone for the treatment of suspected heroin overdose. *Addiction.* 2009 Dec;104 (12):2067–74.

[40] Christenson J, Etherington J, Grafstein E, Innes G, Pennington S, Wanger K, et al. Early discharge of patients with presumed opioid overdose: development of a clinical prediction rule. *Acad. Emerg. Med.* 2000;7 (10):1110–8.

[41] Rudolph S, Jehu G, Nielsen S, Nielsen K, Siersma V, Rasmussen L. Prehospital treatment of opioid overdose in Copenhagen- is it safe to discharge on scene? *Resuscitation.* 2011 Nov;82:1414–8.

[42] Inturrisi CE. Clinical pharmacology of opioids for pain. *Clin. J. Pain.* 2002 Aug;18 (4 Suppl):S3–13.

[43] Inturrisi CE, Max MB, Foley KM, Schultz M, Shin SU, Houde RW. The pharmacokinetics of heroin in patients with chronic pain. *N. Engl. J. Med.* 1984 May 10;310 (19):1213–7.

[44] Zador D, Sunjic S, Darke, S. Heroin-related deaths in New South Wales, 1992: toxicological findings and circumstances. *Med. J. Aust.* 1996 Feb 19;164 (4):204–7.

[45]   United Nations Office on Drugs and Crime, World Health Organization. Opioid overdose: preventing and reducing opioid overdose mortality. New York: United Nations; 2013.

[46]   AMA adopts new policies at annual meeting [Internet]. American Medical Association. 2012 [cited 2015 Jul 27]. Available from: https://www.ama-assn.org/ama/pub/news/news/2012-06-19-ama-adopts-new-policies.page

[47]   American Public Health Association. APHA policy statement LB-11-03 – reducing unintentional prescription drug overdoses [Internet]. American Public Health Association; 2012 [cited 2015 Jul 7]. Available from: http://www.drugpolicy.org/sites/default/files/American%20Public %20Health%20Association%20Statement.pdf

[48]   Wheeler E, Jones T, Gilbert M, Davidson P. Opioid overdose prevention programs providing naloxone to laypersons – United States, 2014. *MMWR Morb Mortal Wkly Rep.* 2015 Jun 19;64 (23):631–5.

[49]   Sporer KA, Firestone J, Isaacs SM. Out-of-hospital treatment of opioid overdoses in an urban setting. *Acad. Emerg. Med.* 1996;3 (7):660–7.

[50]   Ashton H, Hassan Z. Best evidence topic report. Intranasal naloxone in suspected opioid overdose. *Emerg. Med. J.* 2006 Mar;23 (3):221–3.

[51]   Kelly A-M, Kerr D, Dietze P, Patrick I, Walker T, Koutsogiannis Z. Randomised trial of intranasal versus intramuscular naloxone in prehospital treatment for suspected opioid overdose. *Med. J. Aust.* 2005;182 (1):24–7.

[52]   Coffin PO, Sullivan SD. Cost-effectiveness of distributing naloxone to heroin users for lay overdose reversal. *Ann. Intern. Med.* 2013;158 (1):1–9.

[53]   Sporer KA. Strategies for preventing heroin overdose. *Bmj.* 2003;326 (7386):442–4.

[54]   Caplehorn JR, Dalton MS, Haldar F, Petrenas A-M, Nisbet JG. Methadone maintenance and addicts' risk of fatal heroin overdose. *Subst Use Misuse.* 1996;31 (2):177–96.

[55]   Polomeni P, Schwan R. Management of opioid addiction with buprenorphine: French history and current management. *Int. J. Gen. Med.* 2014 Mar 3;7:143–8.

[56]   Ali R. Pharmacologic treatment. ATLAS on substance use (2010) - Resources for the prevention and treatment of substance use disorders [Internet]. Geneva, Switzerland: World Health Organization Press; 2010 [cited 2015 Jul 27]. p. 57–74. Available from: http://cdrwww.who.int/ entity/substance_abuse/activities/msbaltaschthree.pdf

[57] Blieden M. A perspective on the epidemiology of acetaminophen exposure and toxicity in the United States. *Expert Rev. Clin. Pharmacol.* 2014 May;7 (3):341–8.

[58] Larson AM, Polson J, Fontana R, Davern T, Lalani E, Hynan L, et al. Acetaminophen-induced acute liver failure: results of a United States multicenter, prospective study. *Hepatology.* 2005 Dec;42 (6):1364–72.

[59] Department of Justice Drug Enforcement Administration. Schedules of controlled substances: rescheduling of hydrocodone combination products From Schedule III to Schedule II [Docket No. DEA-389]. *Fed. Regist.* 2014 Aug 22;79 (163):49661–82.

[60] Makin A, Williams R. Acetaminophen-induced hepatotoxicity: predisposing factors and treatments. *Adv. Intern. Med.* 1997;42:453–83.

[61] Larson AM. Acetaminophen hepatotoxicity. *Clin. Liver Dis.* 2007 Aug;11 (3):525–48.

[62] Chen W, Koenigs LL, Thompson SJ, Peter RM, Rettie AE, Trager WF, et al. Oxidation of acetaminophen to its toxic quinone imine and nontoxic catechol metabolites by baculovirus-expressed and purified human cytochromes P450 2E1 and 2A6. *Chem. Res. Toxicol.* 1998;11 (4):295–301.

[63] Manyike P, Kharasch E, Kalhorn T, Slattery J. Contribution of CYP2E1 and CYP3A to acetaminophen reactive metabolite formation. *Clin. Pharmacol. Ther.* 2000;67 (3):275–82.

[64] Jollow D, Thorgeirsson S, Potter W, Hashimoto M, Mitchell J. Acetaminophen-induced hepatic necrosis. VI. Metabolic disposition of toxic and nontoxic doses of acetaminophen. *Pharmacology.* 1974;12 (4-5):251–71.

[65] Mitchell J, Jollow D, Potter W, Gillette J, Brodie B. Acetaminophen-induced hepatic necrosis. IV. Protective role of glutathione. *J. Pharmacol. Exp. Ther.* 1974;187 (211-217).

[66] Jaeschke H, Bajt M. Intracellular signaling mechanisms of acetaminophen-induced liver cell death. *Toxicol. Sci.* 2006;89:31–41.

[67] Heard KJ. Acetylcysteine for acetaminophen poisoning. *N. Engl. J. Med.* 2008;359 (3):285–92.

[68] Potter W, Thorgeirsson S, Jollow D, Mitchell J. Acetaminophen-induced hepatic necrosis. V. Correlation of hepatic necrosis, covalent binding and glutathione depletion in hamsters. *Pharmacology.* 1974;12:129–43.

[69] Schmidt L. Age and paracetamol self-poisoning. *Gut.* 2005;54:686–90.

[70] Myers R, Shaheen A, Li B, Dean S, Quan H. Impact of liver disease, alcohol abuse, and unintentional ingestions on the outcomes of

acetaminophen overdose. *Clin. Gastroenterol. Hepatol.* 2008 Aug;6 (8):918–25.

[71] Bray G, Harrison P, O'Grady J, Tredger J, Williams R. Long-term anticonvulsant therapy worsens outcome in paracetamol-induced fulminant hepatic failure. *Hum. Exp. Toxicol.* 1992 Jul;11 (4):265–70.

[72] Chun LJ, Tong MJ, Busuttil RW, Hiatt JR. Acetaminophen hepatotoxicity and acute liver failure. *J. Clin. Gastroenterol.* 2009;43 (4):342–9.

[73] Hodgman MJ, Garrard AR. A review of acetaminophen poisoning. *Crit. Care Clin.* 2012 Oct;28 (4):499–516.

[74] Singer A, Carracio T, Mofenson H. The temporal profile of increased transaminase levels in patients with acetaminophen-induced liver dysfunction. *Ann. Emerg. Med.* 1995 Jul;26 (1):49–53.

[75] Rumack B, Matthew H. Acetaminophen poisoning and toxicity. *Pediatrics.* 1975 Jun;55 (6):871–6.

[76] Nourjah P, Ahmad S, Karwoski C, Willy M. Estimates of acetaminophen (Paracetamol)-associated overdoses in the United States. *Pharmacoepidemiol. Drug Saf.* 2006 Jun 15;15 (6):398–405.

[77] Froberg B, King K, Kurera T, Monte A, Prosser J, Walsh S, et al. Negative predictive value of acetaminophen concentrations within four hours of ingestion. *Acad. Emerg. Med.* 2013 Oct;20 (10):1072–5.

[78] Rumack B. Acetaminophen hepatotoxicity: the first 35 years. *J. Toxicol. Clin. Toxicol.* 2002;40 (1):3–20.

[79] Smilkstein M, Knapp G, Kulig K, Rumack B. Efficacy of oral N-acetylcysteine in the treatment of acetaminophen overdose. Analysis of the national multicenter study (1976 to 1985). *N. Engl. J. Med.* 1988 Dec 15;319 (24):1557–62.

[80] Seifert SA, Kirschner RI, Martin TG, Schrader RM, Karowski K, Anaradian PC. Acetaminophen concentrations prior to 4 hours of ingestion: Impact on diagnostic decision-making and treatment. *Clin. Toxicol.* 2015 Jun 24;1–6.

[81] Brok J, Buckley N, Gluud C. Interventions for paracetamol (acetaminophen) overdose. *Cochrane Database Syst. Rev.* 2006 Apr 19; (2):CD003328.

[82] Holdiness M. Clinical pharmacokinetics of N-acetylcysteine. *Clin. Pharmacokinet.* 1991 Feb;20 (2):123–34.

[83] Slattery J, Wilson J, Kalhorn T, Nelson S. Dose-dependent pharmacokinetics of acetaminophen: evidence of glutathione depletion in humans. *Clin. Pharmacol. Ther.* 1987 Apr;41 (4):413–8.

[84] Prescott L. Treatment of severe acetaminophen poisoning with intravenous acetylcysteine. *Arch. Intern. Med.* 1981;141 (3):386–9.

[85] Harrison P, Keays R, Bray G, Alexander G, Williams R. Improved outcome of paracetamol-induced fulminant hepatic failure by late administration of acetylcysteine. *Lancet.* 1990 Jun 30;335 (8705):1572–3.

[86] Yip L, Dart R, Hurlburt K. Intravenous administration of oral N-acetylcysteine. *Crit. Care Med.* 1998 Jan;26 (1):40–3.

[87] Marbury T, Wang L, Lee C. Hemodialysis of acetaminophen in uremic patients. *Int. J. Artif. Organs.* 1980;3:263–6.

[88] Gosselin S, Juurlink DN, Kielstein JT, Ghannoum M, Lavergne V, Nolin TD, et al. Extracorporeal treatment for acetaminophen poisoning: Recommendations from the EXTRIP workgroup. *Clin. Toxicol.* 2014 Sep;52 (8):856–67.

[89] McPhail M, Kriese S, Heneghan M. Current management of acute liver failure. *Curr. Opin. Gastroenterol.* 31 (3):209–14.

[90] Han M, Hyzy R. Advances in critical care management of hepatic failure and insufficiency. *Crit. Care Med.* 2006 Sep;34 (9 Suppl):S225–31.

[91] Farmer D, Anselmo D, Ghobrial R, Yersiz H, McDiarmid S, Cao C, et al. Liver transplantation for fulminant hepatic failure: experience with than 200 patients over a 17-year period. *Ann. Surg.* 2003 May; 237 (5):666–75.

[92] Benzodiazepines (street names: benzos, downers, nerve pills, tranks) [Internet]. Drug Enforcement Agency, Office of Diversion Control, *Drug & Chemical Evaluation Section.* 2013 [cited 2015 Jul 27]. Available from: http://www.deadiversion.usdoj.gov/drug_chem_info/benzo.pdf

[93] Olfson M, King M, Schoenbaum M. Benzodiazepine use in the Unites States. *JAMA Psychiatry.* 2015;72 (2):136–42.

[94] Sheehan M, Sheehan D, Torres A, Coppola A, Francis E. Snorting benzodiazepines. *Am. J. Drug Alcohol Abuse.* 1991;17 (4):457–68.

[95] Cai R, Crane E, Poneleit K, Paulozzi L. Emergency department visits involving nonmedical use of selected prescription drugs --- United States, 2004--2008. *MMWR Morb Mortal Wkly Rep.* 59 (23):705–9.

[96] Cohen J, Davis S, Furbee P, Sikora R, Tillotson R, Bossarte R. Hospitalizations for poisoning by prescription opioids, sedatives, and tranquilizers. *Am. J. Prev. Med.* 2010;38 (5):517–24.

[97] The CBHSQ report: a day in the life of young adults: substance use facts [Internet]. [cited 2015 Jul 28]. Available from: http://www.samhsa.gov/

data/sites/default/files/CBHSQ-SR168-TypicalDay-2014/CBHSQ-
SR168-TypicalDay-2014.htm
[98] Jones C, Mack K, Paulozzi L. Pharmaceutical overdose deaths, United
States, 2010. *JAMA.* 2013;309 (7):657–9.
[99] Jones J, Mogali S, Comer S. Polydrug abuse: A review of opioid and
benzodiazepine combination use. *Drug Alcohol Depend.* 2012;125 (1-
2):8–18.
[100] Kao M, Zheng P, Mackey S. Trends in benzodiazepine prescritpion and
co-prescription with opioids in the United States, 2002-2009. Phoenix,
AZ; 2014.
[101] U.S Department of Justice. Product No. 2003-L0559-013: prescription
drugs fast facts [Internet]. National Drug Intelligence Center. 2003 [cited
2015 Aug 4]. Available from: http://www.justice.gov/archive/ndic/
pubs5/5140/
[102] Griffin CE, Kaye AM, Bueno FR, Kaye AD. Benzodiazepine
pharmacology and central nervous system-mediated effects. *Ochsner J.*
2013;13 (2):214–23.
[103] Weinbroum A, Flaishon R, Sorkine P, Szold O, Rudik V. A risk-benefit
assessment of flumazenil in the management of benzodiazepine
overdose. *Drug Saf.* 1997; 17 (3):181–96.
[104] Kratz A, Ferraro M, Sluss PM, Lewandrowski KB. Case records of the
Massachusetts General Hospital. Weekly clinicopathological exercises.
Laboratory reference values. *N. Engl. J. Med.* 2004 Oct 7;351
(15):1548–63.
[105] Tietz N (Ed). Clinical guide to laboratory tests. 3rd ed. Philadelphia, PA:
W.B. Saunders; 1995.
[106] Marraffa JM, Cohen V, Howland MA. Antidotes for toxicological
emergencies: A practical review. *Am. J. Health Syst. Pharm.* 2012 Feb
1;69 (3):199–212.
[107] Ward C, Sair M. Oral poisoning: an update. *Contin Educ. Anaesth Crit.
Care Pain.* 2010;10 (1):6–11.
[108] Veldhorst-Janssen NML, Fiddelers AAA, van der Kuy P-HM, Neef C,
Marcus MAE. A review of the clinical pharmacokinetics of opioids,
benzodiazepines, and antimigraine drugs delivered intranasally. *Clin.
Ther.* 2009 Dec;31 (12):2954–87.
[109] Eddey DP, Westcott MJ. "The needle and the damage done": Intra-
arterial temazepam. *Emerg. Med.* 2000; 12 (3):248–52.

[110] Sen S, Chini EN, Brown MJ. Complications after unintentional intra-arterial injection of drugs: Risks, outcomes, and management strategies. *Mayo Clin. Proc.* 2005 Jun; 80 (6):783–95.

[111] Moeller KE, Lee KC, Kissack JC. Urine drug screening: practical guide for clinicians. Mayo Clinic Proceedings [Internet]. Elsevier; 2008 [cited 2015 Jul 27]. p. 66–76. Available from: http://www.sciencedirect.com/science/article/pii/S0025619611611208.

[112] Chyka PA, Seger D, Krenzelok EP, Vale JA, American Academy of Clinical Toxicology, European Association of Poisons Centres and Clinical Toxicologists. Single-dose activated charcoal. *Clin. Toxicol. Phila Pa.* 2005;43 (2):61–87.

[113] Spivey WH. Flumazenil and seizures: analysis of 43 cases. *Clin. Ther.* 1992 Apr;14 (2):292–305.

[114] Flumazenil [Package insert}. Eatontown, NJ: West-Ward Pharmaceuticals; 2011.

In: Drug Overdoses and Alcohol Withdrawal ISBN: 978-1-63483-873-3
Editor: David P. Morales © 2016 Nova Science Publishers, Inc.

Chapter 3

ALCOHOL WITHDRAWAL FROM THE ANGLE OF OXIDATIVE STRESS

Marianna Jung
Department of Pharmacology & Neuroscience,
UNT Health Science Center, Fort Worth, TX, US

ABSTRACT

The prolonged heavy drinking of alcohol (ethanol) often creates brain disorder alcoholism. Individuals with alcoholism experience a difficulty to control the amount of drinking in spite of adverse consequences. In particular, they encounter ethanol withdrawal (EW) syndromes upon a sudden cessation of drinking. The syndromes are largely hyperexcitatory (e.g., tremor, or seizure), due to an increase in excitatory neurotransmitters such as glutamate. Excessive glutamate overly activates its receptors, which in turn increases the entry of Ca^{2+} to the inside of cells and mitochondria. This exacerbates the generation of O_2 derived molecules, reactive oxygen species (ROS). While a moderate amount of ROS has been reported to be beneficial, the high amount of ROS overwhelms antioxidant enzymes and oxidizes cellular components, triggering cell damage, a phenomenon known as oxidative stress. Abundant evidence now indicates that EW stress damages the brain and other organs through mechanisms involving oxidative stress. During EW, ROS in concert with excitatory molecules provoke a wide range of oxidative stress including lipid peroxidation, protein oxidation, DNA oxidation, antioxidant suppression, and redox imbalance towards oxidation. These oxidative events may further interact with each other, amplifying neuronal damage. EW-induced oxidative stress warrants further research, which may ultimately help develop an adjunctive therapy for the successful detoxification of alcoholics who are not benefited by an existing therapy alone.

ABBREVIATIONS

BZDs	Benzodiazepines
ETC	Electron transport complex
EW	Ethanol withdrawal
γ-Amino butyric acid	GABA
8-OHdG	8-hydroxy-deoxyguanosine
iGluR	Ionotropic glutamate receptors
MDA	Malondialdehyde
mGluR	Metabotropic receptors
nNOS	Neuronal NOS
NMDA	N-methyl-D-aspartate
NOS	Nitric oxide synthase
PTP	Mitochondrial membrane permeability transition pore
ROS	Reactive oxygen species
TBARS	Thiobarbituric acid reactive substances

ETHANOL WITHDRAWAL (EW)

Alcoholism is a drinking disorder largely resulting from years of heavy drinking. Patients with alcoholism experience a difficulty to control ethanol consumption in spite of adverse medical and social consequences. The problematic aspect of alcoholism is inferred from a report that alcoholism is a frequent psychiatric diagnosis in patients who commit suicide (Lejoyeux et al., 1994). Symptoms of alcoholism include craving and seeking out alcohol, an inability to control drinking, organ damage, and withdrawal syndromes. Withdrawal syndromes typically occur upon the abrupt termination of long-term heavy drinking and range from psychological symptoms to physical signs. Examples of withdrawal syndromes include anxiety, depression, tremors, irritability, rigidity, hyperactivity, convulsion, delirium tremens (impaired mental status), and even coma or death (Becker 2000; Dissanaike et al., 2006; Yaldizli et al., 2006). Physicians in all areas of medicine frequently encounter managing EW syndromes because alcoholic patients must be detoxified when they are treated for alcohol-related or -unrelated illnesses (Buchsbaum et al., 1985; Graham 1991; Mayo-Smith 1997). In a clinical study, up to 86% of patients admitted for alcohol detoxification have shown some of the EW syndromes (Caetano et al., 1998). Moderate syndromes of EW are considered as problematic as severe ones because they provide a driving force for relapse to avoid the discomforts (Barrett 1985; Covarrubias et al., 2005). Moreover, many alcoholics who attempt to quit drinking repeat the vicious cycle of drinking and abstinence, which increases the intensity of EW syndromes and brain damage (Dahchour and De Witte, 2003) to the point of premature death (Becker and Hale 1993). The premature death can even occur long after complete abstinence (Marmot et al., 1981; Holahan et al., 2010), suggesting that EW induces persistent or permanent brain damage.

THE LIMITATION OF A CURRENT THERAPY FOR EW

Benzodiazepines (BZDs) are a central nervous system (CNS) CNS depressant that potentiates inhibitory neurotransmission by binding the GABA (γ-Amino butyric acid)-BZD receptor complex. BZDs are currently the primary drug of choice for the treatment of EW syndromes (Gold et al., 2007; Sarff and Gold, 2010). However, BZDs have their own dependence liability and are one of the most abused prescription drugs (Justice.gov/DEA). The abuse of BZDs is more frequent in patients who have an alcohol use disorder than other disorders (Mueller et al., 2005), suggesting that alcoholic patients are vulnerable to the risk of BZD dependency. Heavy ethanol consumption for a period of time results in ethanol tolerance, a phenomenon that requires a higher dose of ethanol to achieve the same desired effect of ethanol. Like ethanol, a chronic intake of BZDs creates tolerance. Ethanol shares a common mechanism with BZD by potentiating the activity of GABA/BZD receptors. Because of this overlapped mechanism, alcoholic patients with ethanol tolerance also experience BZD tolerance, requiring a higher dose of BZDs (Book and Myrick, 2005; Gartenmaier et al., 2005). A high dose of BZDs is very sedating and can suppress ventilation (Gillis et al., 1989; Megarbane et al., 2005) to such an extent that emergency medical attention is necessary (Hack et al., 2006). As a step towards developing a better research and therapeutic strategy, we and others have strived to identify the mechanisms by which EW stress provokes neuronal damages. Among a variety of cellular damages and stresses, this review article will focus on the damages associated with oxidative stress.

OXIDATIVE STRESS

Reactive oxygen species (ROS) are a group of unstable species derived from oxygen (O_2) such as hydroxyl radicals (•HO) and superoxide (O_2-), and contain atoms with an unpaired electron. In an attempt to achieve stability, ROS steal electrons from other molecules, and thus, the molecules that lose electrons are oxidized. ROS are produced under physiological conditions as byproducts of oxidation. A moderate level of ROS generation is beneficial by increasing an adaptive strength of cells, called 'positive oxidative stress' (Yan 2014). However, the production of ROS is dramatically increased under pathological conditions, overwhelming endogenous antioxidant enzymes. Such imbalance between a high level of ROS production vs. a low level of antioxidant capacity triggers deleterious molecular events. This type of oxidative stress with adverse consequences will be the main focus of the current review article. Brain is especially sensitive to oxidative stress for a few reasons; brain has a high rate of metabolism that uses O_2 in a relatively small mass compared to other organs (Poon et al., 2004), is rich of redox-active metals that are readily oxidized (Lovell et al., 1998), and has a low level of antioxidant enzymes such as superoxide dismutase and catalase (Khan and Black, 2003). Consequently, brain generates more ROS, which increases its vulnerability to oxidative neuronal damage.

Most, if not all, neurodegenerative disorders involve oxidative stress including those associated with harmful drinking and EW. Ethanol has an intimate relationship with oxidative stress as it directly generates ROS in the process of ethanol metabolism. Ethanol is converted to acetaldehyde by enzymes of alcohol dehydrogenase, cytochrome P450-2E1, and catalase. Acetaldehyde enters mitochondria and is metabolized into acetate. In this process, NADH is simultaneously generated mainly by aldehyde dehydrogenase 2 located in mitochondria. When NADH is converted to NAD^+ by the electron transport complex I, the generation of hydroxyl radicals is increased. Among ROS, hydroxyl radicals are extremely reactive, and cause the oxidation of membrane component, phospholipids (Cheeseman and Slater, 1993). Subsequently, mitochondria lose membrane potential (Hoek et al., 2002) and the fundamental functions of adenosine triphosphate (ATP) production. The oxidative nature of ethanol is important in the central nervous system (CNS) because the CNS consists of a high content of unsaturated (containing double bond) membrane lipid which is a preferred target of both ROS (Hernandez-Munoz et al., 2000) and ethanol (Szelenyi and Brune, 1988). Compared to a direct effect of ethanol on ROS, EW indirectly provokes oxidative stress through excitatory molecules. In some cases, oxidative cellular damage is more severe during EW than ethanol exposure (Follesa et al., 2003; Jung et al., 2009), indicating that EW-related oxidative stress is not merely the residual effect of ethanol exposure.

TARGETS OF OXIDATIVE STRESS DURING EW

Oxidative Stress to Membrane Lipids

The high amount of ROS attacks membrane lipids (Mariet et al., 2012), resulting in lipid radicals that react with O_2 to form peroxyl radicals, an event known as lipid peroxidation. Lipid peroxidation initiates a series of reactions that generate several byproducts, collectively called thiobarbituric acid reactive substances (TBARS). A major example of TBARS is malondialdehyde (MDA) which is the end product of lipid peroxidation and often measured as a marker of oxidative damage to lipid molecules (Huber et al., 1991; Jardine et al., 2002; Grignon et al., 2007).

Clinical studies have documented that ethanol withdrawing patients show oxidative damages to lipid molecules and antioxidant enzyme suppression. Compared to normal individuals, the serum of alcoholic patients during detoxification contained an elevated level of MDA and reduced activity of endogenous antioxidant superoxide dismutase (Lecomte et al., 1994; Peng et al., 2005; Huang et al., 2009). Intriguingly, alcoholic patients with a higher level of MDA suffered from more severe EW syndromes on the first day of detoxification, revealing a strong correlation between MDA level and EW severity (Huang et al., 2009). Even 10 to 15 days after admission for detoxification, alcoholics showed a decreased serum level of antioxidant vitamin E and vitamin A, indicating persistent oxidative damage by EW. The degree of the antioxidant suppression was correlated with the severity of liver failure, brain atrophy, or cerebellar shrinkage (González-Reimers et al., 2014). The increase in oxidative insults and defective antioxidant mechanisms in the alcohol-withdrawn patients are also shown in other human studies. Tsai et al. (1998) have observed a higher level of lipid peroxide and a lower activity of superoxide dismutase in the cerebral spinal fluid of alcohol withdrawn patients than normal individuals. Woźniak et al. (2008) demonstrated that the concentration of TBARS in the blood of alcoholic men was 40% higher before detoxification compared to the control group. The concentration of TBARS was decreased after detoxification but was still higher than that of the control group and remained higher for 6 days after last drinking. The period of 6 days is well beyond time needed for a complete elimination of blood ethanol as alcoholics eliminate blood ethanol at the rate of 30 ± 9 mg% per hour (Winek and Murphy, 1984). This raises an important point that oxidative stress to membrane lipids seen in alcohol withdrawing patients is persistent and may involve EW-specific mechanisms. Animal studies agree with these human studies such that ethanol withdrawn rats show increased plasma levels of TBARS and O_2- (Gonzaga et al., 2015). These studies provide empirical evidence that EW acts as a lasting oxidative stressor to lipid molecules in human and experimental animals.

Oxidative Stress to Protein

The oxidative stress-provoking (pro-oxidant) effects of EW are also seen at the protein level. The significance of protein oxidation is inferred from the reports that the oxidative modification of proteins is often seen in neurodegenerative diseases and aging (Forster et al., 2000; Dalle-Donne et al., 2003). Several markers of protein oxidation have been recognized, including the formation of protein carbonyl, nitrotyrosine, dityrosine, and isoaspartate as well as the loss of protein thiols (Yan 2009). Among these, the measurement of protein carbonyl has been extensively employed by numerous studies (Levine et al., 1990; Forster et al., 2000; Yan et al., 2002). ROS modify proteins (Grimsrud et al., 2008) by the carbonylation of lysine, arginine, proline, and threonine residues of proteins, functionally inactivating the proteins (Amici et al., 1989; Rivett 1989). The amount of protein carbonyl was increased in the blood of ethanol-dependent patients (Mutlu-Turkoglu et al., 2000), and in the liver (Bailey et al., 2001) or pancreas of ethanol exposed rodents (Bailey et al., 2001; Cano et al., 2001; Zhou et al., 2005). Similarly, an increased amount of protein carbonyl was observed in the cerebellum, cortex, and hippocampus of ethanol consuming rats (Jung et al., 2008a). Regarding the effect of EW on protein oxidation, we have shown that protein carbonylation was substantially increased 24 hours after ethanol removal in rats (Jung et al., 2008b). Controversially, abstinent alcoholic patients did not show any increase in protein carbonylation in the cerebrospinal fluid (Tsai et al., 1998). One potential explanation for this discrepancy is a timing effect of EW. For example, carbonyl contents were measured approximately one month after the last ethanol ingestion in the clinical study as compared to one day after the last drinking in our study. As time elapsed, the oxidatively damaged proteins might have been replaced with newly synthesized proteins, resulting in no difference between alcoholic and healthy individuals in that clinical study. Our laboratory has adopted an in vitro model of EW using HT22 cells to assess EW-induced oxidative damage. HT22 cells are derived from a mouse hippocampal cell line and an effective model of oxidative stress. This is because HT22 cells contain a transporter named the glutamate/cystine antiporter that delivers cystine into neuronal cells in the exchange of intracellular glutamate (Tan et al., 1998). Cystine is then used for the biosynthesis of an endogenous antioxidant glutathione. As such, the import of cystine through this transporter is critical to glutathione production as well as protection against oxidative cellular damage. Accordingly, HT22 cellular injury is associated with the insufficient synthesis of glutathione, and consequent oxidative damages (Tan et al., 1998; Zaulyanov et al., 1999). As was the case for in vivo studies, HT22 cells withdrawn for four hours after ethanol exposure for 24 hours encountered an excess generation of ROS and protein carbonylation (Prokai-Tatrai et al., 2009). The consequence of such oxidative stress is detrimental to the point of cell death (Prokai-Tatrai et al., 2009). Protein carbonylation during EW apparently involves excessive glutamate based on a study where glutamate treatment to primary cortical neurons caused an increase in ROS and protein carbonylation (Yi et al., 2008). Taken together, these findings suggest that EW provokes destructive oxidative stress both in in vivo and in vitro conditions through protein oxidation.

Oxidative Stress to DNA

DNA oxidation occurs when the highly reactive hydroxyl radicals react with a nucleotide base, which can cause breaks in DNA strand. This occurs in more than 20 nucleotide bases, most notably C-8 position of the guanine base, generating 8-hydroxy-deoxyguanosine (8-OHdG) (Cooke et al., 2003). 8-OHdG is frequently used to estimate ROS-induced DNA damage (Rehman et al., 1999; Bahar et al., 2007; Schulpis et al., 2007) and has gained much attention because it can produce abnormal products of mutant DNAs (Griffiths et al., 2009). Some studies highlight that the level of this marker reflects a severity of diseases associated with excitatory molecules, for example,

Parkinson's disease (Alam et al., 1997). With regard to oxidative DNA damage by ethanol, Chen et al. (2011) have observed an elevated level of 8-OHdG in the serum of alcoholic patients compared with normal individuals. The increase in 8-OHdG level is significantly correlated with an increase in MDA level as if oxidation occurs in genes of MDA production. In agreement with this human study, brain tissues from animals fed with chronic ethanol show a variety of DNA damages including DNA oxidation, strand breaks, and fragmentation (Cahill et al., 1997, 1999). Whether ethanol-induced oxidative damage to DNA is recoverable seems controversial between animal and human studies. Oxidative DNA damage induced by chronic (30 days) ethanol administration was recovered 3 days after ethanol removal in rats (Guo et al., 2008). Chen et al. (2011) have observed that the level of MDA and 8-OHdG are elevated in the serum of human alcoholics with a drinking history of 11 ± 7.5 years. In Chen's study, the level of MDA was decreased after one week-detoxification but the 8-OHdG levels did not change in the same period. The authors have suggested that a long drinking history of the patients might have been responsible for the persistent elevation of 8-OHdG. Significantly, the increased level of 8-OHdG was better correlated with the severity of EW syndromes than MDA even after confounding variables were normalized (Chen et al., 2011). Should alcoholic patients have a low level of antioxidants to combat oxidative stress, this would provide a favorable milieu to ROS to attack DNA. Indeed, Huang et al. (2009) observed that alcoholic patients suffered from persistently weakened antioxidant activities, including superoxide dismutase and glutathione peroxidase when measured two weeks after detoxification. A rise in the levels of DNA oxidation seen in alcoholic patients could hence be the consequence of not only an increase in oxidative attack to DNA but also a decreased antioxidant activity to repair oxidatively damaged DNA. Since oxidative DNA damages are shown in highly inheritable CNS disorders such as Alzheimer Disease (Mecocci et al., 1998), the prooxidant effect of EW on DNA may thus place alcohol dependent individuals as at high risk for genetic diseases.

EXCITATORY MOLECULES & OXIDATIVE STRESS

Glutamate, a Mediator of EW Stress

Glutamate is the major excitatory neurotransmitter that is most abundant among excitatory neurotransmitters in the CNS. It plays a role in synaptic plasticity (changes in synaptic strength), learning, memory, and maintaining neuronal integrity. However, under pathological conditions, the extracellular glutamate concentration rises sharply to an mM range. This induces the excessive or prolonged activation of glutamate receptors, initiating the process of neuronal death, a phenomenon known as excitotoxicity (Coyle and Puttfarcken, 1993; al Qatari et al., 2001; Lipton 2007). The rise in the concentration of extracellular glutamate plays a more critical role in excitotoxicity than intracellular concentration. Glutamate inside the cells is relatively inactive (Dan 2012) and glutamate receptors can be activated by glutamate binding to them from the outside. Glutamate at its high extracellular level is believed to be a central player in the pathogenesis of many human neurodegenerative disorders such as ischemic stroke, epilepsy, Alzheimer disease, and Huntington's disease (Meldrum et al., 1992; Chapman, 1998; Nakao and Brundin, 1998; Lipton, 1999; Revett et al., 2013; Ribeiro et al., 2014).

EW stress is initiated by a sudden removal of neuro-inhibitory ethanol, and thus, renders a rebound increase in excitatory neurotransmissions. A body of studies has shown that the extracellular level of glutamate is elevated and over-activates its receptor in ethanol withdrawing humans and experimental animals (Tsai et al., 1998; Dahchour and De Witte, 1999, Dahchour and De Witte, 2003). In fact, the upregulation of glutamatergic neurotransmissions has been recognized as a hallmark of EW and the mechanisms underlying EW syndromes (Tsai et al., 1998; Nagy et al., 2001; Prendergast et al., 2004). There are two major classes of glutamate receptors: metabotropic and ionotropic receptor. Glutamate binds the metabotropic glutamate receptors (mGluR) which requires secondary messenger molecules such as G protein, thereby initiating the cascade of intracellular signaling in the activated neuron. At least 8 different types of mGluR (mGluR1 - mGluR8) have been reported based on the structure and activity of the receptors. Glutamate also binds the ionotropic glutamate receptors (iGluR) and opens a pore (channel) of iGluR. iGluR are further divided into three subtypes according to their selective agonists: 2-amino-3-hydroxy-5-methyl-4-isoxazolepropionic acid (AMPA), N-methyl-D-aspartate (NMDA), and kainic acid (Watkins et al., 1990; Nakanishi et al., 1992; Sommer et al., 1992). The hyperactivation of iGluR subsequently opens postsynaptic ion channels, thereby increasing the entry of Na^+, K^+, and Ca^{2+} to the inside of neurons and leading to excitatory neuronal disorders (Finn and Crabbe 1997; Lipton 1999). Among three types of iGluR, NMDA receptors have been particularly recognized as a mediator of EW-induced excitatory stress in part due to their high Ca^{2+} permeability (Nagy 2008).

Studies on EW stress indicate the involvement of both mGluR and iGluR in the pathogenesis of EW. Kumar et al. (2013) have shown that the antagonist of mGluR5 ameliorates EW-induced anxiety in rats. The antagonists of mGlu1 and mGlu5 also attenuate EW-induced audiogenic seizures in rats (Kotlinska et al., 2011). The iGluR as a mediator of EW stress has been demonstrated in studies where the administration of NMDA or NMDA antagonists to ethanol withdrawn animals results in an increase (Sanna et al., 1993) or a decrease (Faingold et al., 2000) in seizure activity, respectively. In addition to mGluR and iGluR, the glutamate/cystine antiporter appears to mediate EW stress. We have documented that EW suppresses the viability of HT22 cells (Jung et al., 2009) that lack or minimally contain iGluR; thus, the EW-induced HT22 cellular injury is unlikely through iGluR (Zaulyanov et al., 1999). As mentioned earlier, HT22 cells contain the glutamate/cystine antiporter, raising a possibility that the cytotoxic effects of EW at least partly result from the damaged antiporter, and a concomitant reduction in endogenous antioxidant capacity (Tan et al., 1998). The advantage of EW stress acting through both types of glutamate receptors as well as the glutamate/cystine antiporter may readily overload glutamate signals to neurons, provoking oxidative damage.

Excitatory Molecules, Oxidative Mediators of EW Stress

The over-stimulation of glutamate receptors has been suggested as a main mediator of intracellular oxidative stress (Coyle and Puttfarcken, 1993; Kim and Pae, 1996; Facchinetti et al., 1998). Upon the activation of glutamate receptors, the excessive level of Ca^{2+} enters cells and mitochondria, impeding the function of electron transport complex (ETC) ETC and ATP generation. The malfunction of mitochondria exacerbates the production of ROS and triggers the cascade of cell death pathways (Vergun et al., 2001). A clinical significance of these oxidative events is inferred from a study where human alcoholics with more severe EW syndromes show a higher level of glutamate and MDA (Tsai et al., 1998). Homocysteine is another excitatory molecule that acts as an endogenous agonist at the glutamate binding site of the NMDA receptor. Upon binding to its receptor, homocysteine potentiates excitatory postsynaptic potentials (Lipton et al., 1997) and increases intracellular Ca^{2+} concentration (Kim and Pae, 1996). Alcoholic patients who suffered from withdrawal seizures had significantly higher levels of homocysteine than alcoholic patients who did not develop seizures (Bleich et al., 2000). These observations led Bleich et al. (2000) to propose the plasma level of homocysteine as a predictor of seizures among the various signs of EW syndromes. Homocysteine may have a functional relationship with oxidative stress; the level of both homocysteine and MDA were elevated in the serum of alcoholic patients during the first three days of withdrawal (Bleich et al., 2000). Bleich et al. (2000) have suggested that ROS mediate neuronal damage induced by excitatory molecules, and hereby cause brain shrinkage and neuronal death in the alcohol withdrawing patients. All these studies support the existence of a mechanistic link between the upregulation of excitatory molecules and EW-induced oxidative damage.

CA^{2+} AND OXIDATIVE STRESS

Ca^{2+} mediates communication between electrical signaling involving an action potential and chemical signaling involving neurotransmitters. Action potential is a rapid change in the electrical potential (mv) of membranes for cell to cell communication. During normal physiological conditions, action potential reaches axon terminal, depolarizes the axon membrane, and subsequently opens voltage-gated Na^+ channels. Na^+ ions then enter the cell, depolarize the presynaptic membrane, and open Ca^{2+} channels. This allows the entry of Ca^{2+} ions to the inside of cells. To reiterate, excessive glutamate induces the hyperactivation of iGluR that provide a channel for Ca^{2+} entry to cells. This in turn provokes mitochondrial Ca^{2+} overload, and ruptures mitochondrial membranes. The idea that Ca^{2+} mediates the excitatory effect of EW stress is supported by previous studies where Ca^{2+} signal evoked by a glutamate receptor agonist was enhanced by EW in cultured primary Purkinje neurons of rat (Netzeband et al., 2002). The level of Ca^{2+} in the synaptosomal membranes obtained from rat brain was increased during EW even to a greater degree than during ethanol exposure (Virmani et al., 1985). Increased Ca^{2+} current and Ca^{2+} entry to the inside of cells are followed by seizure occurrence during EW (N'Gouemo et al., 2003). Due to such a critical role of excessive Ca^{2+} in cell damage, cells have endogenous protective machinery to tightly control the level of intracellular Ca^{2+}. Parvalbumin is a Ca^{2+} binding protein and its binding to Ca^{2+} reduces the level of free, non-bound, intracellular Ca^{2+}. Mutant mice lacking parvalbumin show similar signs to EW syndromes such as epileptic seizures (Caillard et al., 2000; Vecellio et al., 2000). By comparison, parvalbumin-containing neurons survive temporal lobe epilepsy (Sloviter 1989; Ince et al., 1993). These studies have prompted us to measure the level of parvalbumin during EW. We observed that the level of parvalbumin was significantly decreased 24 hours after the removal of an ethanol diet for 5 weeks in rats (Rewal et al., 2005). It is thus plausible that EW-induced parvalbumin suppression increases intracellular Ca^{2+}, contributing to excitatory neuronal damage. A potential involvement of oxidative stress in this process is supported by a study where the activation of the O_2- producing enzyme led to the loss of parvalbumin containing neurons in prefrontal cortex (Behrens and Sejnowski, 2009). This effect of oxidative insults was not seen after treatment with glutamate receptor antagonist ketamine, suggesting that glutamate mediates oxidative-damage to the parvalbumin containing neurons. A direct effect of parvalbumin on cellular oxidative stress was discovered by Permyakov et al. (2014) who observed the conformation-dependent oxidation of the parvalbumin molecule. In another word, parvalbumin helps the reduction (opposite to oxidation) of other molecules by oxidizing itself, reflecting an antioxidant activity of parvalbumin. This series of Ca^{2+} events support the hypothesis that the excessive level of intracellular and mitochondrial Ca^{2+} mediates EW-induced oxidative cellular damage.

MITOCHONDRIA

Mitochondria and Oxidative Stress

How Ca^{2+} mediates oxidative stress during EW is postulated to involve mitochondria. The primary function of mitochondria is to produce cellular energy as a form of adenosine triphosphate (ATP) through a series of mitochondrial enzyme complexes, the electron transport complex (ETC). ETC consists of ETCI, II, III, and IV that are embedded in the inner mitochondrial membranes. Electrons are transferred across the ETC with the aid of the electron carriers. Simultaneously, protons (H^+) are pumped out of mitochondria, creating the electrochemical gradient between the inner and outer membranes of mitochondria. Protons outside of the mitochondria flow passively back into the mitochondrial matrix through a pore associated with the ATP synthase, providing a force to generate ATP. ROS are produced as byproducts of ETC activities, placing mitochondria at a high risk for oxidative damage. ROS production was increased when SH-SY5Y cells (human neuroblastoma derived) were treated with ETC II inhibitor malonate (Fernandez-Gomez et al., 2005), suggesting that a damage to ETC exacerbates the mitochondrial production of ROS. Excessive ROS alter mitochondrial proteins, impeding mitochondrial function as seen in in vitro studies using human cells: H_2O_2 treatment caused the oxidation of mitochondrial proteins in conjunction with ATP depletion in cultured human fibroblasts (Miyoshi et al., 2006) and human lens epithelial cells (Wang et al., 2003). When ATP levels fall, the action of sodium/potassium (Na^+/K^+) exchange pump is diminished as this pump uses ATP. Under normal conditions, the negative potential (-70 mv) of resting cellular membrane is maintained by Na^+/K^+ pump that pumps three sodium ions out of cells in exchange with two potassium ions into the cells. Therefore, the diminished function of this pump renders the cell membrane potential drifting toward more depolarized (toward positive) potentials, which allows more action potentials, and neuronal firing. The fast-firing of neurons increases the probability of opening voltage-dependent sodium and Ca^{2+} channels in response to excitatory stimuli (Dutta 2011). The depolarization by bioenergetic deficit causes glutamate even at a non-toxic concentration to become lethal (Novelli et al., 1988).

EW Damages Mitochondria

Convincing evidence now indicates that EW stress produces severe mitochondrial damage. The cellular energy status of cultured granular cells is decreased by EW with concurrent mitochondrial membrane swelling and mitochondrial respiratory suppression (Follesa et al., 2003). The mitochondrial damage induced by EW may be attributed to oxidative stress. EW induces the excessive level of intracellular Ca^{2+}, subsequently overloading mitochondria with Ca^{2+}. The high amount of Ca^{2+} in mitochondria suppresses cellular energy generation (Kristian et al., 1998), increases ROS generation (Hansson et al., 2008), and provokes excitotoxicity (Budd and Nicholls, 1996). Our previous study has shown that the amount of protein oxidation is higher in mitochondrial fractions than whole cell lysates obtained from ethanol withdrawn rats (Jung et al., 2008b)., This indicatesing that EW stress renders mitochondria particularly vulnerable to oxidative stress. In favor of this view, withdrawal for 24 hours after four days of ethanol exposure elevated mitochondrial ROS generation and lipid peroxidation in rat liver (Rouach et al., 1983).

Since EW increases glutamate neurotransmission, studies on glutamate are relevant to the interplay between EW and oxidative mitochondrial damage. NMDA infusion into the lateral ventricle induces ruptured mitochondria in rats (Dietrich et al., 1992), suggesting that NMDA mediates the mitochondrial damage. The glutamate antagonist treatment decreased the mitochondrial production of MDA in cerebellum (Reddy et al., 2011), suggesting that glutamate mediates the lipid peroxidation in mitochondria. Mitochondria use glutamate as a form of its metabolite (α-ketoglutarate) to drive the tricarboxylic acid (TCA) cycle that provides electrons for mitochondrial ATP synthesis. In the TCA cycle, α-ketoglutarate is converted to succinyl CoA by α-ketoglutarate dehydrogenase with the simultaneous conversion of NAD^+ to NADH. The higher ratio of $NADH/NAD^+$ produces the higher rate of H_2O_2 production (Tretter and Adam-Vizi (2004), indicating the pro-oxidant property of NADH (Figure 1). Tretter and Adam-Vizi (2004) made intriguing observations about this enzyme in synaptosomes prepared from the brain cortex of guinea pigs: isolated α-ketoglutarate dehydrogenase increases the mitochondrial generation of ROS (H_2O_2), and the catalytic function is activated by Ca^{2+}. The authors suggested that the activation of this enzyme significantly contributes to oxidative stress in the mitochondria. The apparent interplay between glutamate and Ca^{2+} may mediate oxidative damage to mitochondria challenged by EW.

Mitochondrial Membrane Permeability Transition Pore (PTP)

The role of mitochondria in maintaining redox balance reportedly involves membrane permeability that is regulated by a group of proteins called the mitochondrial membrane permeability transition pore (PTP). PTP controls permeability to electrolytes, nucleotides and metabolic substrates, all of which are essential for ATP production. PTP is believed to be minimally composed of adenine nucleotide translocase (ANT), mitochondrial creatine kinase, voltage dependent anion channel, and cyclophilin D (Connern and Halestrap, 1994; Dolder et al., 2001; Lipskaya et al., 2001; Halestrap and Brennerb, 2003). A prolonged opening of PTP diffuses water and electrolytes across the mitochondrial membranes, which causes the collapse of mitochondrial membrane potential (ψm) (Stuart, 2002). Accordingly, ψm is often measured as a marker of PTP. One way that Ca^{2+} enters mitochondria is through PTP. The regulatory function of PTP proteins is impeded when PTP encounters the massive amount of Ca^{2+} entry to mitochondria (Halestrap and Brennerb, 2003). Consequently, mitochondria face membrane swelling, ETC malfunction (Yan et al., 2002; Halestrap and Brennerb, 2003), and ROS over-production. Yan et al. (2002) have reported that PTP component proteins are a direct target of oxidative damage. They observed that the protein carbonyl content of

ANT1 (heart muscle isoform of ANT) is increased in the absence of heat shock factor 1 with an antioxidant property. They also observed that the oxidative damage to ANT1 increased PTP opening, suggesting that PTP opening and oxidative stress mutually exacerbate each other's condition. Our prior study has demonstrated that EW provokes mitochondrial membrane swelling and ψm collapse (Jung et al., 2009). This effect of EW concurs with an increase in ROS generation.

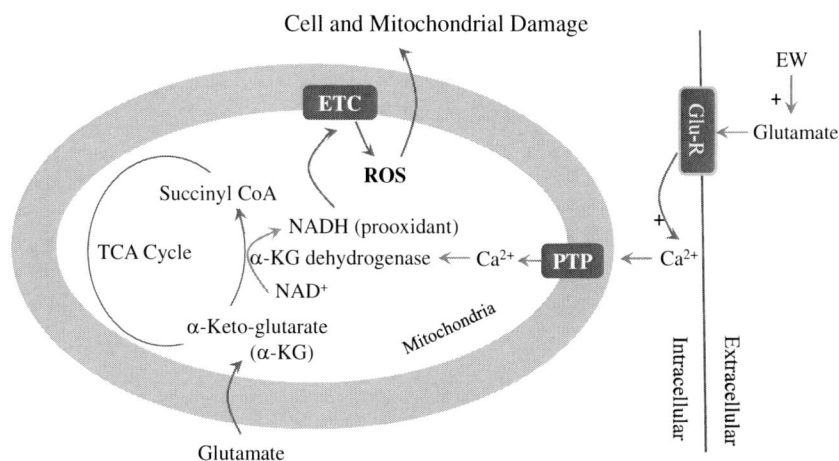

Figure 1. How EW-induced glutamate provokes mitochondrial ROS generation. Upon EW, the extracellular level of glutamate is increased. Glutamate activates its receptors (Glu-R), in turn provoking the excessive entry of Ca^{2+} to cells, and subsequently to mitochondria through PTP. Ca^{2+} activates TCA enzyme α-ketoglutarate (α-KG) dehydrogenase with the simultaneous production of prooxidant NADH. An increase in NADH may hyper-activate ETC activity, exacerbating ROS production. Moreover, the excessive Ca^{2+} entry to mitochondria through PTP results in prolonged PTP opening, which damages mitochondrial membrane components including ETC. This also exacerbates ROS production. "+" indicates activation/upregulation.

Excessive ROS alter the stability, conformation, activity, and function of the PTP proteins, resulting in prolonged PTP opening (Yan et al., 2002; Vyssokikh et al., 2003). Based on these studies, we tested whether antioxidants protect mitochondrial membranes from EW stress (Jung et al., 2009). We used three compounds with ROS scavenging activities: 17β-estradiol, butylated hydroxytoluene, and ZYC26, an analogue of 17β-estradiol.

ZYC26 has shown 10-fold higher antioxidant potency than 17β-estradiol in the HT22 cell model of EW (Jung et al., 2006). ZYC26 contains an adamantyl group at the C2 position of A-ring. This structural configuration enhances the stability of the adjacent phenoxyl radical, which is an essential element of ROS scavenging activity (Prokai et al., 2007). We measured the mitochondrial membrane swelling of ethanol withdrawn HT22 cells with the expectation that ZYC26 would show a greater protection against membrane swelling than other two compounds. Unexpectedly, all three compounds mitigated the mitochondrial membrane swelling with a similar degree of potency (Jung et al., 2009). This highlights an important point that oxidative stress is a part of, not a sole mechanism of mitochondrial and neuronal damage.

REACTIVE NITROGEN SPECIES (RNS)

ROS interact with RNS such as nitric oxide (NO) and NO-derived free radicals that act as molecular messengers in the CNS. NO is synthesized from l-arginine by a nitric oxide synthase (NOS) using O_2 and NADPH (reduced nicotinamide adenine dinucleotide phosphate) as a cofactor (Andrew and Bernd, 1999; Bian and Murad, 2003; West and Tseng, 2011). There are three major isoforms of NOS; neuronal NOS (nNOS), endothelial NOS (eNOS) and inducible NOS (iNOS) based on the activity or tissue type in which they were first described. NOS requires Ca^{2+} and Ca^{2+}-modulating protein calmodulin for their activity but whether all three or only certain (eNOS and nNOS) isoforms require Ca^{2+} seems under investigation. NO rapidly reacts with O_2- to yield the peroxynitrite anion (ONOO-). NO or ONOO- reacts with other molecules present in high concentrations to form adducts that might be responsible for protein oxidation, DNA damage (Dawson and Dawson, 1996), and apoptotic cell death (Martin et al., 2011). Two decades ago, different laboratories simultaneously discovered the localization of NOS in mitochondria (Bates et al., 1995; Kobzik et al., 1995; Bates et al., 1996; Frandsen et al., 1996). Whether mitochondrial NOS is different from three major isoforms of NOS or which isoform is located in mitochondria appears to be under debate. This mitochondrially-localized NOS can be a threat to mitochondria as it produces harmful NO or ONOO- inside the mitochondria, readily damaging redox balance (Figure 2).

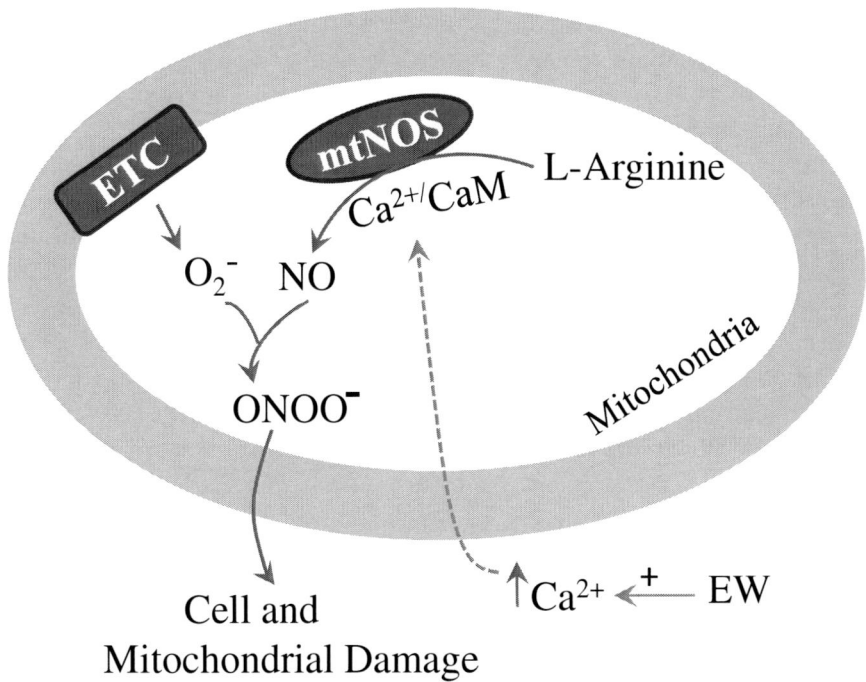

Figure 2. How EW-induced excessive Ca^{2+} increases ROS-RNS interaction. The interaction between O_2- and NO generates harmful molecule ONOO-. The synthesis of NO requires NOS and its cofactors such as Ca^{2+} and calmodulin (CaM). Mitochondrial Ca^{2+} overload during EW may increase the activity of NOS. This event may be facilitated by the presence of mitochondrially located NOS (mtNOS). "+" indicates activation/upregulation.

Like ROS, the neurotoxic effect of NO involves glutamate receptors. The activation of NMDA receptors increases the amount and synthesis of NOS (Garthwaite et al., 1989; Parkash et al., 2010). NOS activity is increased when brain is challenged with excitatory molecule kainic acid (Swamy et al., 2009). The high activity of NOS is accompanied by the decreased activity of glutamine synthetase (Swamy et al., 2009) that converts glutamate to glutamine. The activity loss of glutamine synthetase increases the availability of glutamate, which may result in excitotoxic cell death. A pharmacological inhibition of nNOS significantly reduces lesions produced by focal ischemia (Dalkara et al., 1994) and intrastriatal injections of NMDA (Schulz et al., 1995). Mice lacking the nNOS gene are protected from NMDA-mediated excitotoxicity (Dawson et al., 1996), suggesting a reciprocal interaction between NOS and NMDA underlying excitotoxicity. Ca^{2+} contributes to the functional interaction between NOS and NMDA based on a study where the activation of NMDA receptor by glutamate causes an influx of Ca^{2+} into neurons leading to the activation of NOS (Southam et al., 1991).

Previous studies assessed the role of NOS in EW syndromes by treating ethanol withdrawn rats with a NOS inhibitor (nitroindazole) and monitoring the degree of EW syndromes. The severity of EW syndromes was significantly reduced in ethanol withdrawn rats treated with nitroindazole compared with vehicle-treated ethanol withdrawn rats (Uzbay et al., 1997; Adams et al., 1998). Consistent with this animal study, serum obtained from alcoholic patients who were undergoing EW have shown the elevated level of RNS (nitrite) and malondialdehyde (MDA) (Yuksel et al., 2005). How RNS mediates EW syndromes is an open question but postulated to involve Ca^{2+}. For example, NO causes an increase in Ca^{2+} flux into neurons as a consequence of NMDA receptor stimulation by glutamate (Uzbay and Oglesby, 2001).

P38 AND OXIDATIVE STRESS

Protein kinases attach phosphate (p) to proteins, largely activating the phosphorylated proteins. p38 belongs to the superfamily of mitogen-activated protein kinases (MAPK) that are activated by mitogen, a substance that induces cell division. MAPK phosphorylate other proteins as well as they are phosphorylated (activated) by their upstream kinases (MAPK kinase). MAPK function as a critical mediator of signal transduction for gene expression, cell growth, and death. p38 is also known as a stress-activated protein kinase as it is activated by a variety of stresses such as inflammatory cytokines (help move cells towards inflammation sites), oxidative stress, hypoxia, and ischemia (Cuadrado and Nebreda, 2010). At least four isoforms of p38 have been identified so far: p38α, β, γ, and δ. Among these, p38α is particularly responsive to stressful stimuli (Han et al., 1994) including oxidative stress (Gutiérrez-Uzquiza et al., 2012). p38α and p38β are highly expressed in brain areas of cerebral cortex, hippocampus, and cerebellum (Lee et al., 2000). These brain areas are known to mediate psychomotor (pertinent to cognition and movement) functions as well as a major target of drinking-related brain damage. Although p38 activation promotes cell survival (Nemoto et al., 1998; Roulston et al., 1998), many studies agree that stress-activated kinases mediate programmed cell death, apoptosis. Apoptosis is a normal process in which certain cells need to die at some point of their lifespan for a better maintenance of other cells. However, apoptosis is increased to a harmful level when neuronal cells are exposed to a high level of excitatory amino acids, O_2- , NO (Sastry and Rao, 2000), and other stressful stimuli. O'Donnell et al. (2000) have observed that the over-activation of p38 occurs in the liver of aged rats treated with H_2O_2, suggesting a cross-talk between p38 and ROS. A pro-apoptotic protein p53 may mediate the cross-talk such that p38α phosphorylated the serine residue of p53 when liver cells were exposed to H_2O_2 (Xiao et al., 2015). A functional interaction between p38 and oxidative stress is further shown by Giraldo et al. (2014) using vitamin E analogue, trolox. They measured the active form of p38 (p-p38) in the primary culture of cortical neurons treated with a neurotoxin β-amyloid peptide (Aβ) in the presence or absence of trolox. They found that trolox-treatment prevented p38 activation induced by Aβ. This in vitro study was confirmed by an in vivo study where transgenic mice with Alzheimer's diseaseAD genes show an increase in the hippocampal p38 activation in a manner that was prevented by feeding animals with a vitamin E-containing diet. These studies underpin the role of oxidative stress in p38 activation, and p38 activation in oxidative stress, mediating cell damage.

p38 is implicated in excitotoxicity (Kawasaki et al., 1997) as evidenced by p38 activation induced by a high dose of glutamate (Suh et al., 2007). We have demonstrated that the activity and protein level of active p38 are increased in ethanol withdrawn rats (Jung et al., 2011). The increase in p38 in ethanol withdrawn rats is in line with a body of evidence that p38 activation plays an important role in excitotoxic and neurodegenerative processes (Cao et al., 2004). NMDA treatment induces the death of AF5 cell (rat mesencephalic cell line) accompanied by an increase in phosphorylated p38 and ROS generation (Chen et al., 2005). Similarly, Park et al. (2004) treated cortical neurons with NMDA and observed an increase in ROS generation, which was prevented by p38 inhibitor cotreatment. Later, a similar observation was made by Tian et al. (2014); when PC12 cells were treated with glutamate, ROS formation was increased in a manner that was attenuated by p38 inhibition. Together with p38 activation induced by oxidative stress (Giraldo et al., 2014), these studies support the mutually activating effect of p38 and oxidative stress underlying excitatory cellular damage. Mitochondria appear to be associated with this pathway. SH-SY5Y neuroblastoma cells treated with the inhibitor of ETCII (malonate) showed an increase in the levels of MDA, an event that was reduced by a p38 inhibitor SKF86002 (Gomez-Lazaro et al., 2007).

References	EW-induced oxidative pathway
	EW
Tsai et al., 1998; Prendergast et al., 2004	↓
	Glutamate release
Sanna et al., 1993; Kumar et al., 2013	↓
	Glutamate receptor activation
Kumar et al., 2013	↓
	Ca^{2+} entry to cell
Kristian et al., 1998	↓
	Ca^{2+} overload to Mitochondria
Halestrap and Brennerb, 2003	↓
	PTP prolonged opening
Pepe 2000; Yan et al., 2002	↓
	ETC damage
Fernandez-Gomez et al., 2005	↓
	ROS production
Halestrap and Brennerb, 2003	↓
Woźniak et al., 2008; Huang et al., 2009 Jung et al., 2008; Prokai-Tatrai et al., 2009 Chen et al., 2011	Lipid peroxidation, Protein carbonylation, DNA oxidation

Figure 3. A pathway of oxidative damage during EW.
EW stress increases the extracellular glutamate level and activates its receptors. This provokes the excessive entry of Ca^{2+} to cells and overloads mitochondria with Ca^{2+}. When the large amount of Ca^{2+} enters mitochondria through PTP, it overwhelms the capacity of PTP, resulting in prolonged PTP opening. The prolonged PTP opening adversely alters mitochondrial membrane components including ETC and exacerbates ROS production. The ROS then evoke oxidative damage to membrane lipid, protein, and DNA, ultimately resulting in cell damage. This diagram illustrates only one way direction to simplify the pathway.

The same research group conducted a series of other experiments using SH-SY5Y cells to test the interaction between ROS and p38. For example, Fernandez-Gomez (2005) and Gomez-Lazaro et al. (2007) have demonstrated that malonate treatment generates ROS, activates p38, and induces the translocation of a proapoptotic protein BAX to mitochondria. All of these effects of malonate were reduced by treating cells with an antioxidant vitamin E. These phenomena are strikingly similar to those associated with EW such as an increase in ROS, p38 activation, the mitochondrial level of BAX, mitochondrial membrane permeability, and apoptotic neuronal damage. The similarity between the effects of malonate and EW on p38 leads to the hypothesis that p38 mediates the prooxidant effects of EW through mitochondrial factors. A series of findings from our and others' laboratories support this hypothesis. For example, EW-induced ROS generation is reduced by a p38 inhibitor treatment (Jung et al., 2011). Bax translocation to mitochondria is reportedly essential for cell death (Ghatan et al., 2000), and the translocation is induced by malonate (Gomez-Lazaro et al. (2007) but prevented by p38 inhibitor SKF86002 (Gomez-Lazaro et al., 2007). Moreover, cells treated with NO donor sodium nitroprusside encountered Bax translocation to the mitochondria, resulting in cell death (Ghatan et al., 2000). Again, a NO donor cotreatment with a p38 inhibitor protected against BAX translocation and cell death (Ghatan et al., 2000). The authors suggest that p38 activation is necessary for NO-induced neuronal death. Although some of these studies are not directly related to EW stress, they support the idea that p38 is linked to oxidative stress through mitochondria-damaging molecules.

CONCLUSION

Oxidative stress is a common mechanism underlying many neurodegenerative disorders including EW syndromes. EW syndromes are typically hyperexcitatory as they are initiated by the removal of neuro-inhibitory ethanol and a rebound increase in excitatory molecules. EW provokes oxidative stress through excitatory molecules such as glutamate and Ca^{2+} (Figure 3). The concept of oxidative stress as a mediator of neurotoxicity of EW has been accepted by various oxidative molecular changes induced by EW including ROS generation, protein oxidation, lipid oxidation, DNA oxidation, and antioxidant enzymatic suppression. These oxidative events in concert with excitatory molecules further interact with each other, amplifying neuronal damages. Understanding how excitatory molecules interplay with ROS and oxidized cellular components may provide an important mechanistic insight into the research and therapeutic strategies for managing EW stress.

ACKNOWLEDGMENT

This work was supported by UNTHSC IAADR grant. I wish to thank Daniel Metzger for editorial assistance.

REFERENCES

Adams, M. L. & Cicero, T. J. (1998). Alcohol intoxication and withdrawal: the role of nitric oxide. *Alcohol, 16*, 153-158.

al Qatari, M., Khan, S., Harris, B. & Littleton, J. (2001). Acamprosate is neuroprotective against glutamate-induced excitotoxicity when enhanced by ethanol withdrawal in neocortical cultures of fetal rat brain. *Alcohol Clin Exp Res, 25*, 1276-1283.

Alam, Z. I., Jenner, A, Daniel, S. E., Lees, A. J., Cairns, N., Marsden, C. D., Jenner, P. & Halliwell, B. (1997). Oxidative D. N.A damage in the Parkinsonian brain: an apparent selective increase in 8-hydroxyguanine levels in substantia nigra. *J Neurochem, 69*, 1196-1203.

Allen, M., Zou, F., Chai, H. S., Younkin, C. S., Miles, R., Nair, A. A., Crook, J. E., Pankratz, V. S., Carrasquillo, M. M., Rowley, C. N., Nguyen, T., Ma, L., Malphrus, K. G., Bisceglio, G., Ortolaza, A. I., Palusak, R., Middha, S., Maharjan, S., Georgescu, C., Schultz, D., Rakhshan, F., Kolbert, C. P., Jen, J., Sando, S. B., Aasly, J. O., Barcikowska, M., Uitti, R. J., Wszolek, Z. K., Ross, O. A., Petersen, R. C., Graff-Radford, N. R., Dickson, D. W., Younkin, S. G. & Ertekin-Taner, N. (2012). Glutathione S-transferase omega genes in Alzheimer and Parkinson disease risk, age-at-diagnosis and brain gene expression: an association study with mechanistic implications. *Mol Neurodegener, 7*, 13.

Amici, A., Levine, R. L., Tsai, L. & Stadtman, E. R. (1989). Conversion of amino acid residues in proteins and amino acid homopolymers to carbonyl derivatives by metal-catalyzed oxidation reactions. *J Biol Chem, 264*, 3341-3346.

Andrew, P. J. & Mayer, B. (1999). Enzymatic function of nitric oxide synthases. *Cardiovasc Res, 43*, 521-531.

Bahar, G., Feinmesser, R., Shpitzer, T., Popovtzer, A. & Nagler, R. M. (2007). Salivary analysis in oral cancer patients: DN. A and protein oxidation, reactive nitrogen species, and antioxidant profile. *Cancer, 109*, 54-59.

Bailey, S. M., Patel, V. B., Young, T. A., Asayama, K. & Cunningham, C. C. (2001). Chronic ethanol consumption alters the glutathione/glutathione peroxidase-1 system and protein oxidation status in rat liver. *Alcohol Clin Exp Res*, 25, 726-733.

Barrett, R. (1985). Behavioral approaches to individual differences in substance abuse., in *Determinants of substance abuse: biological, pyschological, and environmental factors.* (Galizio ed). 125-174, New York.

Bates, T. E., Loesch, A., Burnstock, G. & Clark, J. B. (1995). Immunocytochemical evidence for a mitochondrially located nitric oxide synthase in brain and liver. *Biochem Biophys Res Commun*, 213, 896-900.

Bates, T. E., Loesch, A, Burnstock, G. & Clark, J. B. (1996). Mitochondrial nitric oxide synthase: a ubiquitous regulator of oxidative phosphorylation? *Biochem Biophys Res Commun*, 218, 40-44.

Becker, H. C. (2000). Animal models of alcohol withdrawal. *Alcohol Res Health*, 24, 105-113.

Becker, H. C. & Hale, R. L. (1993). Repeated episodes of ethanol withdrawal potentiate the severity of subsequent withdrawal seizures: an animal model of alcohol withdrawal "kindling." *Alcohol Clin Exp Res*, 17, 94-98.

Behrens, M. M. & Sejnowski, T. J. (2009). Does schizophrenia arise from oxidative dysregulation of parvalbumin-interneurons in the developing cortex? *Neuropharmacology*, 57, 193-200.

Bian, K. & Murad, F. (2003). Nitric oxide (NO).--biogeneration, regulation, and relevance to human diseases. *Front Biosci*, 8, d264-278.

Book, S. W. & Myrick, H. (2005). Novel anticonvulsants in the treatment of alcoholism. *Expert Opin Investig Drugs*, 14, 371-376.

Buchsbaum, D. G., Buchanan, R. G., Poses, R. M., Schnoll, S. H. & Lawton, M. J. (1992). Physician detection of drinking problems in patients attending a general medicine practice. *J Gen Intern Med*, 7, 517-521.

Budd, S. L. & Nicholls, D. G. (1996). Mitochondria, calcium regulation, and acute glutamate excitotoxicity in cultured cerebellar granule cells. *J Neurochem*, 67, 2282-2291.

Caetano, R., Clark, C. L. & Greenfield, T. K. (1998). Prevalence, trends, and incidence of alcohol withdrawal symptoms: analysis of general population and clinical samples. *Alcohol Health Res World*, 22, 73-79.

Cahill, A., Stabley, G. J., Wang, X. & Hoek, J. B. (1999). Chronic ethanol consumption causes alterations in the structural integrity of mitochondrial DNA in aged rats. *Hepatology*, 30, 881-888.

Cahill, A., Wang, X. & Hoek, J. B. (1997). Increased oxidative damage to mitochondrial D. N.A following chronic ethanol consumption. *Biochem Biophys Res Commun*, *235*, 286-290.

Caillard, O., Moreno, H., Schwaller, B., Llano, I., Celio, M. R. & Marty, A. (2000). Role of the calcium-binding protein parvalbumin in short-term synaptic plasticity. *Proc Natl Acad Sci U S A*, *97*, 13372-13377.

Cano, M. J., Ayala, A., Murillo, M. L. & Carreras, O. (2001). Protective effect of folic acid against oxidative stress produced in 21-day postpartum rats by maternal-ethanol chronic consumption during pregnancy and lactation period. *Free Radic Res*, *34*, 1-8.

Cao, J., Semenova, M. M., Solovyan, V. T., Han, J., Coffey, E. T. & Courtney, M. J. (2004). Distinct requirements for p38alpha and c-Jun N-terminal kinase stress-activated protein kinases in different forms of apoptotic neuronal death. *J Biol Chem*, *279*, 35903-35913.

Chapman, A. G. (1998). Glutamate receptors in epilepsy. *Prog Brain Res*, *116*, 371-383.

Cheeseman, K. H. & Slater, T. F. (1993). An introduction to free radical biochemistry. *Br Med Bull*, *49*, 481-493.

Chen, C. H., Pan, C. H., Chen, C. C. & Huang, M. C. (2011). Increased oxidative D. N.A damage in patients with alcohol dependence and its correlation with alcohol withdrawal severity. *Alcohol Clin Exp Res*, *35*, 338-344.

Chen, J., Errico, S. L. & Freed, W. J. (2005). Reactive oxygen species and p38 phosphorylation regulate the protective effect of Delta9-tetrahydrocannabinol in the apoptotic response to NMDA. *Neurosci Lett*, *389*, 99-103.

Connern, C. P. & Halestrap, A. P. (1994). Recruitment of mitochondrial cyclophilin to the mitochondrial inner membrane under conditions of oxidative stress that enhance the opening of a calcium-sensitive non-specific channel. *Biochem J*, *302* **(Pt 2)**.321-324.

Cooke, M. S., Evans, M. D., Dizdaroglu, M. & Lunec, J. (2003). Oxidative DNA damage: mechanisms, mutation, and disease. *FASEB J 17*, 1195-1214.

Covarrubias, M. Y., Khan, R. L., Vadigepalli, R., Hoek J. B. & Schwaber, J. S. (2005). Chronic alcohol exposure alters transcription broadly in a key integrative brain nucleus for homeostasis: the nucleus tractus solitarius. *Physiol Genomics*, *24*, 45-58.

Coyle, J. T. & Puttfarcken, P. (1993). Oxidative stress, glutamate, and neurodegenerative disorders. *Science*, *262*, 689-695.

Cuadrado, A. & Nebreda, A. R. (2010). Mechanisms and functions of p38 MAPK. signalling. *Biochem J*, *429*, 403-417.

Dahchour, A. & De Witte, P. (1999). Effect of repeated ethanol withdrawal on glutamate microdialysate in the hippocampus. *Alcohol Clin Exp Res*, *23*, 1698-1703.

Dahchour, A. & De Witte, P. (2003a). Effects of acamprosate on excitatory amino acids during multiple ethanol withdrawal periods. *Alcohol Clin Exp Res*, *27*, 465-470.

Dahchour, A. & De Witte, P. (2003b). Excitatory and inhibitory amino acid changes during repeated episodes of ethanol withdrawal: an in vivo microdialysis study. *Eur J Pharmacol*, *459*, 171-178.

Dalkara, T., Yoshida, T., Irikura, K. & Moskowitz, M. A. (1994). Dual role of nitric oxide in focal cerebral ischemia. *Neuropharmacology*, *33*, 1447-1452.

Dalle-Donne, I., Giustarini, D., Colombo, R., Rossi, R. & Milzani, A. (2003). Protein carbonylation in human diseases. *Trends Mol Med*, *9*, 169-176.

Dawson, V. L. & Dawson, T. M. (1996a). Nitric oxide actions in neurochemistry. *Neurochem Int*, *29*, 97-110.

Dawson, V. L. & Dawson, T. M. (1996b). Nitric oxide neurotoxicity. *J Chem Neuroanat*, *10*, 179-190.

Dawson, V. L., Kizushi, V. M., Huang, P. L., Snyder, S. H. & Dawson, T. M. (1996). Resistance to neurotoxicity in cortical cultures from neuronal nitric oxide synthase-deficient mice. *J Neurosci*, *16*, 2479-2487. Justice.gov (2011). Benzodiazepines. http://www.dea.gov/druginfo /factsheets.shtml

Dietrich, W. D., Halley, M., Alonso, O., Globus, M. Y. & Busto, R. (1992). Intraventricular infusion of N-methyl-D-aspartate. 2. Acute neuronal consequences. *Acta Neuropathol*, *84*, 630-637.

Dissanaike, S., Halldorsson, A., Frezza, E. E. & Griswold, J (2006). An ethanol protocol to prevent alcohol withdrawal syndrome. *J Am Coll Surg*, *203*, 186-191.

Dolder, M., Wendt, S. & Wallimann, T. (2001). Mitochondrial creatine kinase in contact sites: interaction with porin and adenine nucleotide translocase, role in permeability transition and sensitivity to oxidative damage. *Biol Signals Recept*, *10*, 93-111.

Dutta, R. & Trapp, B. D. (2011). Mechanisms of neuronal dysfunction and degeneration in multiple sclerosis. *Prog Neurobiol*, *93*, 1-12.

Facchinetti, F., Dawson, V. L. & Dawson, T. M. (1998). Free radicals as mediators of neuronal injury. *Cell Mol Neurobiol*, *18*, 667-682.

Faingold, C., Li, Y. & Evans, M. S. (2000). Decreased GABA and increased glutamate receptor-mediated activity on inferior colliculus neurons in vitro are associated with susceptibility to ethanol withdrawal seizures. *Brain Res*, *868*, 287-295.

Fernandez-Gomez, F. J., Galindo, M. F., Gomez-Lazaro, M., Yuste V. J., Comella, J. X., Aguirre, N. & Jordan, J. (2005). Malonate induces cell death via mitochondrial potential collapse and delayed swelling through an R. O.S-dependent pathway. *Br J Pharmacol*, *144*, 528-537.

Finn, D. A. & Crabbe, J. C. (1997). Exploring alcohol withdrawal syndrome. *Alcohol Health Res World*, *21*, 149-156.

Follesa, P., Mancuso, L., Biggio, F., Mostallino, M. C., Manca, A., Mascia, M. P., Busonero, F., Talani, G., Sanna, E. & Biggio, G. (2003). Gamma-hydroxybutyric acid and diazepam antagonize a rapid increase in GABA.(A). receptors alpha(4). subunit mRNA abundance induced by ethanol withdrawal in cerebellar granule cells. *Mol Pharmacol*, *63*, 896-907.

Forster, M. J., Sohal, B. H. & Sohal, R. S. (2000). Reversible effects of long-term caloric restriction on protein oxidative damage. *J Gerontol A Biol Sci Med Sci*, *55*, B522-529.

Frandsen, U., Lopez-Figueroa, M. & Hellsten, Y. (1996). Localization of nitric oxide synthase in human skeletal muscle. *Biochem Biophys Res Commun*, *227*, 88-93.

Gartenmaier, A., Pelzer, E. & Soyka, M. (2005). Treatment of alcohol withdrawal syndrome with combined carbamazepine and tiapride in a patient with probable sleep apnoe syndrome. *Pharmacopsychiatry*, *38*, 96-98.

Garthwaite, J., Garthwaite, G., Palmer, R. M. & Moncada, S. (1989). N. M.D. A. receptor activation induces nitric oxide synthesis from arginine in rat brain slices. *Eur J Pharmacol*, *172*, 413-416.

Ghatan, S., Larner, S., Kinoshita, Y., Hetman, M., Patel, L., Xia, Z., Youle R. J. & Morrison, R. S. (2000). p38 MAP kinase mediates bax translocation in nitric oxide-induced apoptosis in neurons. *J Cell Biol*, *150*, 335-347.

Gillis, R. A., Namath, I. J., Easington, C., Abrahams, T. P., Guidotti, A., Quest, J. A., Hamosh, P. & Taveira da Silva, A. M. (1989). Drug interaction with gamma-aminobutyric acid/benzodiazepine receptors at the ventral surface of the medulla results in pronounced changes in cardiorespiratory activity. *J Pharmacol Exp Ther*, *248*, 863-870.

Giraldo, E., Lloret, A., Fuchsberger, T. & Vina, J. (2014). Abeta and tau toxicities in Alzheimer's are linked via oxidative stress-induced p38 activation: protective role of vitamin E. *Redox Biol, 2*, 873-877.

Gold, J. A., Rimal, B, Nolan, A. & Nelson L. S. (2007). A strategy of escalating doses of benzodiazepines and phenobarbital administration reduces the need for mechanical ventilation in delirium tremens. *Crit Care Med, 35*, 724-730.

Gomez-Lazaro, M., Galindo, M. F., Melero-Fernandez de Mera, R. M., Fernandez-Gomez, F. J., Concannon, C. G., Segura, M. F., Comella, J. X., Prehn, J. H. & Jordan, J. (2007). Reactive oxygen species and p38 mitogen-activated protein kinase activate Bax to induce mitochondrial cytochrome c release and apoptosis in response to malonate. *Mol Pharmacol, 71*, 736-743.

Gonzaga, N. A., Mecawi, A. S., Antunes-Rodrigues, J., De Martinis, B. S., Padovan, C. M. & Tirapelli, C. R. (2015). Ethanol withdrawal increases oxidative stress and reduces nitric oxide bioavailability in the vasculature of rats. *Alcohol, 49*, 47-56.

Gonzalez-Reimers, E., Fernandez-Rodriguez, C. M., Candelaria Martin-Gonzalez, M., Hernandez-Betancor, I., Abreu-Gonzalez, P., Jose de la Vega-Prieto, M., Elvira-Cabrera, O. & Santolaria-Fernandez, F. (2014). Antioxidant vitamins and brain dysfunction in alcoholics. *Alcohol Alcohol, 49*, 45-50.

Graham, A. W. (1991). Screening for alcoholism by life-style risk assessment in a community hospital. *Arch Intern Med, 151*, 958-964.

Griffiths, L. M., Doudican, N. A., Shadel, G. S. & Doetsch, P. W. (2009). Mitochondrial D. N.A oxidative damage and mutagenesis in Saccharomyces cerevisiae. *Methods Mol Biol, 554*, 267-286.

Grignon, S. & Chianetta, J. M. (2007). Assessment of malondialdehyde levels in schizophrenia: a meta-analysis and some methodological considerations. *Prog Neuropsychopharmacol Biol Psychiatry, 31*, 365-369.

Grimsrud, P. A., Xie, H., Griffin, T. J. & Bernlohr, D. A. (2008). Oxidative stress and covalent modification of protein with bioactive aldehydes. *J Biol Chem, 283*, 21837-21841.

Guo, L., Yang, J. Y. & Wu, C. F. (2008). Oxidative DNA damage induced by ethanol in mouse peripheral leucocytes. *Basic Clin Pharmacol Toxicol, 103*, 222-227.

Gutierrez-Uzquiza, A., Arechederra, M., Bragado, P., Aguirre-Ghiso, J. A. & Porras, A .(2012). p38alpha mediates cell survival in response to oxidative stress via induction of antioxidant genes: effect on the p70S6K pathway. *J Biol Chem*, *287*, 2632-2642.

Hack, J. B., Hoffmann, R. S. & Nelson, L. S. (2006). Resistant alcohol withdrawal: does an unexpectedly large sedative requirement identify these patients early? *J Med Toxicol*, *2*, 55-60.

Halestrap, A. P. & Brenner, C. (2003). The adenine nucleotide translocase: a central component of the mitochondrial permeability transition pore and key player in cell death. *Curr Med Chem*, *10*, 1507-1525.

Han, J., Lee, J. D., Bibbs, L. & Ulevitch, R. J. (1994). AMAP kinase targeted by endotoxin and hyperosmolarity in mammalian cells. *Science*, *265*, 808-811.

Hansson, M J., Mansson, R., Morota, S., Uchino, H., Kallur, T., Sumi, T., Ishii, N., Shimazu, M., Keep, M. F., Jegorov, A & Elmer, E (2008). Calcium-induced generation of reactive oxygen species in brain mitochondria is mediated by permeability transition. *Free Radic Biol Med*, *45*, 284-294.

Hernandez-Munoz, R., Montiel-Ruiz, C. & Vazquez-Martinez, O. (2000). Gastric mucosal cell proliferation in ethanol-induced chronic mucosal injury is related to oxidative stress and lipid peroxidation in rats. *Lab Invest*, *80*, 1161-1169.

Hoek, J. B., Cahill, A. & Pastorino, J. G. (2002). Alcohol and mitochondria: a dysfunctional relationship. *Gastroenterology*, *122*, 2049-2063.

Holahan, C. J., Schutte, K. K., Brennan, P. L., Holahan, C. K., Moos, B. S. & Moos, R. H. (2010). Late-life alcohol consumption and 20-year mortality. *Alcohol Clin Exp Res*, *34*, 1961-1971.

Huang, M. C., Chen, C. H., Peng, F. C., Tang, S. H. & Chen, C. C. (2009). Alterations in oxidative stress status during early alcohol withdrawal in alcoholic patients. *J Formos Med Assoc*, *108*, 560-569.

Huber, W., Kraupp-Grasl, B., Esterbauer, H. & Schulte-Hermann, R. (1991). Role of oxidative stress in age dependent hepatocarcinogenesis by the peroxisome proliferator nafenopin in the rat. *Cancer Res*, *51*, 1789-1792.

Ince, P., Stout, N., Shaw, P., Slade, J., Hunziker, W., Heizmann, C. W. & Baimbridge, K. G. (1993). Parvalbumin and calbindin D-28k in the human motor system and in motor neuron disease. *Neuropathol Appl Neurobiol*, *19*, 291-299.

Jardine, D., Antolovich, M., Prenzler, P. D. & Robards, K. (2002). Liquid chromatography-mass spectrometry (LC-MS). investigation of the thiobarbituric acid reactive substances (TBARS). reaction. *J Agric Food Chem*, *50*, 1720-1724.

Jung, M. E., Ju, X, Simpkins, J. W., Metzger, D. B., Yan, L. J. & Wen, Y. (2011). Ethanol withdrawal acts as an age-specific stressor to activate cerebellar P38 kinase. *Neurobiol Aging, 32*, 2266-2278.

Jung, M. E., Simpkins, J. W., Wilson, A. M., Downey, H. F. & Mallet, R. T. (2008a). Intermittent hypoxia conditioning prevents behavioral deficit and brain injury in ethanol-withdrawn rats. *J Appl Physiol, (1985). 105*, 510-517.

Jung, M. E., Wilson, A. M., Ju, X., Wen, Y., Metzger, D. B. & Simpkins, J. W. (2009). Ethanol withdrawal provokes opening of the mitochondrial membrane permeability transition pore in an estrogen-preventable manner. *J Pharmacol Exp Ther, 328*, 692-698.

Jung, M. E., Wilson, A. M. & Simpkins, J. W. (2006). A nonfeminizing estrogen analog protects against ethanol withdrawal toxicity in immortalized hippocampal cells. *J Pharmacol Exp Ther, 319*, 543-550.

Jung, M. E., Yan, L. J., Forster, M. J. & Simpkins, J. W. (2008b). Ethanol withdrawal provokes mitochondrial injury in an estrogen preventable manner. *J Bioenerg Biomembr, 40*, 35-44.

Kawasaki, H., Morooka, T., Shimohama, S., Kimura, J., Hirano, T., Gotoh, Y. & Nishida, E. (1997). Activation and involvement of p38 mitogen-activated protein kinase in glutamate-induced apoptosis in rat cerebellar granule cells. *J Biol Chem, 272*, 18518-18521.

Khan, J. Y. & Black, S. M. (2003). Developmental changes in murine brain antioxidant enzymes. *Pediatr Res, 54*, 77-82.

Kim, W. K. & Pae, Y. S. (1996). Involvement of N-methyl-d-aspartate receptor and free radical in homocysteine-mediated toxicity on rat cerebellar granule cells in culture. *Neurosci Lett, 216*, 117-120.

Kobzik, L., Stringer, B., Balligand, J. L., Reid, M. B. & Stamler, J. S. (1995). Endothelial type nitric oxide synthase in skeletal muscle fibers: mitochondrial relationships. *Biochem Biophys Res Commun, 211*, 375-381.

Kotlinska, J. H., Bochenski, M. & Danysz, W. (2011). The role of group I mGlu receptors in the expression of ethanol-induced conditioned place preference and ethanol withdrawal seizures in rats. *Eur J Pharmacol, 670*, 154-161.

Kristian, T. & Siesjo, B. K. (1998). Calcium in ischemic cell death. *Stroke, 29*, 705-718.

Kumar, J., Hapidin, H., Bee, Y. T. & Ismail, Z. (2013). Effects of the mGluR5 antagonist MPEP on ethanol withdrawal induced anxiety-like syndrome in rats. *Behav Brain Funct, 9*, 43.

Lecomte, E., Herbeth, B., Pirollet, P., Chancerelle, Y., Arnaud, J., Musse, N., Paille, F., Siest, G. & Artur, Y. (1994). Effect of alcohol consumption on blood antioxidant nutrients and oxidative stress indicators. *Am J Clin Nutr, 60*, 255-261.

Lee, S. H., Park, J., Che, Y., Han, P. L. & Lee, J. K. (2000). Constitutive activity and differential localization of p38alpha and p38beta MAPKs in adult mouse brain. *J Neurosci Res, 60*, 623-631.

Lejoyeux, M., Leon, E. & Rouillon, F. (1994). [Prevalence and risk factors of suicide and attempted suicide]. *Encephale, 20*, 495-503.

Levine, R. L., Garland, D., Oliver, C. N., Amici, A., Climent, I., Lenz, A. G., Ahn, B. W., Shaltiel, S. & Stadtman, E. R. (1990). Determination of carbonyl content in oxidatively modified proteins. *Methods Enzymol, 186*, 464-478.

Lipskaya, T. Y. (2001). Mitochondrial creatine kinase: properties and function. *Biochemistry (Mosc). 66*, 1098-1111.

Lipton, P. (1999). Ischemic cell death in brain neurons. *Physiol Rev, 79*, 1431-1568.

Lipton, S. A. (2007). Pathologically-activated therapeutics for neuroprotection: mechanism of NMDA receptor block by memantine and S-nitrosylation. *Curr Drug Targets, 8*, 621-632.

Lipton, S. A., Kim, W. K., Choi, Y. B., Kumar, S., D'Emilia, D. M., Rayudu, P. V., Arnelle, D. R. & Stamler, J. S. (1997). Neurotoxicity associated with dual actions of homocysteine at the N-methyl-D-aspartate receptor. *Proc Natl Acad Sci U S A, 94*, 5923-5928.

Lovell, M. A., Robertson, J. D., Teesdale, W. J., Campbell, J. L. & Markesbery, W. R. (1998). Copper, iron and zinc in Alzheimer's disease senile plaques. *J Neurol Sci, 158*, 47-52.

Marmot, M. G., Rose, G. & Shipley, M. J. (1981). Alcohol and mortality. *Lancet, 1*, 1159.

Martin, L. J., Adams, N. A., Pan, Y., Price, A. & Wong, M. (2011). The mitochondrial permeability transition pore regulates nitric oxide-mediated apoptosis of neurons induced by target deprivation. *J Neurosci, 31*, 359-370.

Mayo-Smith, M. F. (1997). Pharmacological management of alcohol withdrawal. A meta-analysis and evidence-based practice guideline. American Society of Addiction Medicine Working Group on Pharmacological Management of Alcohol Withdrawal. *JAMA 278*, 144-151.

Mecocci, P., Polidori, M. C., Ingegni, T., Cherubini, A., Chionne, F., Cecchetti, R. & Senin, U. (1998). Oxidative damage to D. N.A in lymphocytes from A. D. patients. *Neurology*, *51*, 1014-1017.

Megarbane, B., Lesguillons, N., Galliot-Guilley, M., Borron, S. W., Trout, H., Decleves, X., Risede, P., Monier, C., Boschi, G. & Baud, F. J. (2005). Cerebral and plasma kinetics of a high dose of midazolam and correlations with its respiratory effects in rats. *Toxicol Lett*, *159*, 22-31.

Meldrum, B. S., Swan, J. H., Leach, M. J., Millan, M. H., Gwinn, R., Kadota, K., Graham, S. H., Chen, J. & Simon, R. P. (1992). Reduction of glutamate release and protection against ischemic brain damage by BW 1003C87. *Brain Res*, *593*, 1-6.

Miyoshi, N., Oubrahim, H., Chock, P. B. & Stadtman, E. R. (2006). Age-dependent cell death and the role of ATP in hydrogen peroxide-induced apoptosis and necrosis. *Proc Natl Acad Sci U S A*, *103*, 1727-1731.

Mueller, T. I., Pagano, M. E., Rodriguez, B. F., Bruce, S. E., Stout, R. L. & Keller, M. B. (2005). Long-term use of benzodiazepines in participants with comorbid anxiety and alcohol use disorders. *Alcohol Clin Exp Res*, *29*, 1411-1418.

Mutlu-Turkoglu, U., Dogru-Abbasoglu, S., Aykac-Toker, G., Mirsal, H., Beyazyurek, M. & Uysal, M. (2000). Increased lipid and protein oxidation and D. N.A damage in patients with chronic alcoholism. *J Lab Clin Med*, *136*, 287-291.

N'Gouemo, P. & Morad, M. (2003). Ethanol withdrawal seizure susceptibility is associated with upregulation of L- and P-type Ca2+ channel currents in rat inferior colliculus neurons. *Neuropharmacology*, *45*, 429-437.

Nagy, J. (2008). Alcohol related changes in regulation of NMDA receptor functions. *Curr Neuropharmacol*, *6*, 39-54.

Nagy, J., Muller, F. & Laszlo, L. (2001). Cytotoxic effect of alcohol-withdrawal on primary cultures of cortical neurones. *Drug Alcohol Depend*, *61*, 155-162.

Nakanishi, S. (1992). Molecular diversity of glutamate receptors and implications for brain function. *Science*, *258*, 597-603.

Nakao, N. & Brundin, P. (1998). Neurodegeneration and glutamate induced oxidative stress. *Prog Brain Res*, *116*, 245-263.

Nemoto, S., Xiang, J., Huang, S. & Lin, A. (1998). Induction of apoptosis by S. B.202190 through inhibition of p38beta mitogen-activated protein kinase. *J Biol Chem*, *273*, 16415-16420.

Netzeband, J. G., Schneeloch, J. R., Trotter, C., Caguioa-Aquino, J. N. & Gruol, D. L. (2002). Chronic ethanol treatment and withdrawal alter A

CPD-evoked calcium signals in developing Purkinje neurons. *Alcohol Clin Exp Res, 26*, 386-393.

Novelli, A., Reilly, J. A., Lysko, P. G. & Henneberry, R. C. (1988). Glutamate becomes neurotoxic via the N-methyl-D-aspartate receptor when intracellular energy levels are reduced. *Brain Res, 451*, 205-212.

O'Donnell, E., Vereker, E. & Lynch, M. A. (2000). Age-related impairment in L. T.P is accompanied by enhanced activity of stress-activated protein kinases: analysis of underlying mechanisms. *Eur J Neurosci, 12*, 345-352.

Park, J. Y., Kim, E. J., Kwon, K. J., Jung, Y. S., Moon, C. H., Lee, S. H. & Baik, E. J. (2004). Neuroprotection by fructose-1,6-bisphosphate involves ROS alterations via p38 MAPK/ERK. *Brain Res, 1026*, 295-301.

Parkash, J., d'Anglemont de Tassigny, X., Bellefontaine, N., Campagne, C., Mazure, D., Buee-Scherrer, V. & Prevot, V. (2010). Phosphorylation of N-methyl-D-aspartic acid receptor-associated neuronal nitric oxide synthase depends on estrogens and modulates hypothalamic nitric oxide production during the ovarian cycle. *Endocrinology, 151*, 2723-2735.

Peng, F. C., Tang, S. H., Huang, M. C., Chen, C. C., Kuo., T. L. & Yin, S. J. (2005). Oxidative status in patients with alcohol dependence: a clinical study in Taiwan. *J Toxicol Environ Health A, 68*, 1497-1509.

Permyakov, S. E., Kazakov, A. S., Avkhacheva, N. V. & Permyakov, E. A. (2014). Parvalbumin as a metal-dependent antioxidant. *Cell Calcium, 55*, 261-268.

Poon, H. F., Calabrese, V., Scapagnini, G. & Butterfield, D. A. (2004). Free radicals and brain aging. *Clin Geriatr Med, 20*, 329-359.

Prendergast, M. A., Harris, B. R., Mullholland, P. J., Blanchard, J. A., 2nd, Gibson, D. A., Holley, R. C. & Littleton, J. M. (2004). Hippocampal CA.1 region neurodegeneration produced by ethanol withdrawal requires activation of intrinsic polysynaptic hippocampal pathways and function of N-methyl-D-aspartate receptors. *Neuroscience, 124*, 869-877.

Prokai-Tatrai, K., Prokai, L., Simpkins, J. W. & Jung, M. E. (2009). Phenolic compounds protect cultured hippocampal neurons against ethanol-withdrawal induced oxidative stress. *Int J Mol Sci, 10*, 1773-1787.

Prokai, L. & Simpkins, J. W. (2007). Structure-nongenomic neuroprotection relationship of estrogens and estrogen-derived compounds. *Pharmacol Ther, 114*, 1-12.

Reddy, N. R., Krishnamurthy, S., Chourasia, T. K., Kumar, A. & Joy, K. P. (2011). Glutamate antagonism fails to reverse mitochondrial dysfunction in late phase of experimental neonatal asphyxia in rats. *Neurochem Int, 58*, 582-590.

Rehman, A., Nourooz-Zadeh, J., Moller, W., Tritschler, H., Pereira, P., & Halliwell, B. (1999). Increased oxidative damage to all D. N.A bases in patients with type II diabetes mellitus. *FEBS Lett, 448*, 120-122.

Revett, T. J., Baker, G. B., Jhamandas, J & Kar, S. (2013). Glutamate system, amyloid ss peptides and tau protein: functional interrelationships and relevance to Alzheimer disease pathology. *J Psychiatry Neurosci, 38*, 6-23.

Rewal, M., Wen, Y., Wilson, A., Simpkins, J. W. & Jung, M. E. (2005). Role of parvalbumin in estrogen protection from ethanol withdrawal syndrome. *Alcohol Clin Exp Res, 29*, 1837-1844.

Ribeiro, F. M., Hamilton, A., Doria, J. G., Guimaraes, I. M., Cregan, S. P. & Ferguson, S. S. (2014). Metabotropic glutamate receptor 5 as a potential therapeutic target in Huntington's disease. *Expert Opin Ther Targets, 18*, 1293-1304.

Rivett, A. J. (1989). High molecular mass intracellular proteases. *Biochem J, 263*, 625-633.

Roulston, A., Reinhard, C., Amiri, P. & Williams, L. T. (1998). Early activation of c-Jun N-terminal kinase and p38 kinase regulate cell survival in response to tumor necrosis factor alpha. *J Biol Chem, 273*, 10232-10239.

Sanna, E., Serra, M., Cossu, A., Colombo, G., Follesa, P., Cuccheddu, T., Concas, A. & Biggio, G. (1993). Chronic ethanol intoxication induces differential effects on GABAA and NMDA receptor function in the rat brain. *Alcohol Clin Exp Res, 17*, 115-123.

Sarff, M. & Gold, J. A. (2010). Alcohol withdrawal syndromes in the intensive care unit. *Crit Care Med, 38*, S494-501.

Sastry, P. S. & Rao, K. S. (2000). Apoptosis and the nervous system. *J Neurochem, 74*, 1-20.

Schulpis, K. H., Lazaropoulou, C., Vlachos, G. D., Partsinevelos, G. A., Michalakakou, K., Gavrili, S., Gounaris, A., Antsaklis, A. & Papassotiriou, I. (2007). Maternal-neonatal 8-hydroxy-deoxyguanosine serum concentrations as an index of D. N.A oxidation in association with the mode of labour and delivery. *Acta Obstet Gynecol Scand, 86*, 320-326.

Schulz, J. B., Matthews, R. T., Jenkins, B. G., Ferrante, R. J., Siwek, D., Henshaw, D. R., Cipolloni, P. B., Mecocci, P., Kowall, N. W., Rosen, B. R. et al. (1995). Blockade of neuronal nitric oxide synthase protects against excitotoxicity in vivo. *J Neurosci, 15*, 8419-8429.

Sloviter, R. S. (1989). Calcium-binding protein (calbindin-D28k). and parvalbumin immunocytochemistry: localization in the rat hippocampus with specific reference to the selective vulnerability of hippocampal neurons to seizure activity. *J Comp Neurol, 280*, 183-196.

Sommer, B. & Seeburg, P. H. (1992). Glutamate receptor channels: novel properties and new clones. *Trends Pharmacol Sci, 13*, 291-296.

Southam, E., East, S. J. & Garthwaite, J. (1991). Excitatory amino acid receptors coupled to the nitric oxide/cyclic GMP pathway in rat cerebellum during development. *J Neurochem, 56*, 2072-2081.

Stuart, R. (2002). Insertion of proteins into the inner membrane of mitochondria: the role of the Oxa1 complex. *Biochim Biophys Acta, 1592*, 79-87.

Suh, H. W., Kang, S. & Kwon, K. S. (2007). Curcumin attenuates glutamate-induced HT22 cell death by suppressing MAP kinase signaling. *Mol Cell Biochem, 298*, 187-194.

Swamy, M., Sirajudeen, K. N. & Chandran, G. (2009). Nitric oxide (NO)., citrulline-NO cycle enzymes, glutamine synthetase, and oxidative status in kainic acid-mediated excitotoxicity in rat brain. *Drug Chem Toxicol, 32*, 326-331.

Szelenyi, I. & Brune, K. (1988). Possible role of oxygen free radicals in ethanol-induced gastric mucosal damage in rats. *Dig Dis Sci, 33*, 865-871.

Tan, S., Wood, M. & Maher, P. (1998). Oxidative stress induces a form of programmed cell death with characteristics of both apoptosis and necrosis in neuronal cells. *J Neurochem, 71*, 95-105.

Tayfun, Uzbay, I. & Oglesby, M. W. (2001). Nitric oxide and substance dependence. *Neurosci Biobehav Rev, 25*, 43-52.

Tian, X., Sui, S., Huang, J., Bai, J. P., Ren, T. S. & Zhao, Q. C. (2014). Neuroprotective effects of Arctium lappa L. roots against glutamate-induced oxidative stress by inhibiting phosphorylation of p38, JNK and ERK 1/2 MAPKs in PC12 cells. *Environ Toxicol Pharmacol 38*, 189-198.

Tretter, L. & Adam-Vizi, V. (2004). Generation of reactive oxygen species in the reaction catalyzed by alpha-ketoglutarate dehydrogenase. *J Neurosci, 24*, 7771-7778.

Tsai, G. E., Ragan, P., Chang, R., Chen, S., Linnoila, V. M. & Coyle, J. T. (1998). Increased glutamatergic neurotransmission and oxidative stress after alcohol withdrawal. *Am J Psychiatry, 155*, 726-732.

Uzbay, I. T., Erden, B. F., Tapanyigit, E. E. & Kayaalp, S. O. (1997). Nitric oxide synthase inhibition attenuates signs of ethanol withdrawal in rats. *Life Sci, 61*, 2197-2209.

Vecellio, M., Schwaller, B., Meyer, M., Hunziker, W. & Celio, M. R. (2000). Alterations in Purkinje cell spines of calbindin D-28 k and parvalbumin knock-out mice. *Eur J Neurosci, 12*, 945-954.

Vergun, O., Sobolevsky, A. I., Yelshansky, M. V., Keelan, J., Khodorov, B. I. & Duchen, M. R. (2001). Exploration of the role of reactive oxygen species in glutamate neurotoxicity in rat hippocampal neurones in culture. *J Physiol, 531*, 147-163.

Virmani, M., Majchrowicz, E., Swenberg, C. E., Gangola, P. & Pant, H. C. (1985). Alteration in calcium-binding activity in synaptosomal membranes from rat brains in association with physical dependence upon ethanol. *Brain Res, 359*, 371-374.

Vyssokikh, M. Y. & Brdiczka, D. (2003). The function of complexes between the outer mitochondrial membrane pore (V. D.A. C.). and the adenine nucleotide translocase in regulation of energy metabolism and apoptosis. *Acta Biochim Pol, 50*, 389-404.

Wang, X., Simpkins, J. W., Dykens, J. A. & Cammarata, P. R. (2003). Oxidative damage to human lens epithelial cells in culture: estrogen protection of mitochondrial potential, ATP, and cell viability. *Invest Ophthalmol Vis Sci, 44*, 2067-2075.

Watkins, J. C., Krogsgaard-Larsen, P. & Honore, T. (1990). Structure-activity relationships in the development of excitatory amino acid receptor agonists and competitive antagonists. *Trends Pharmacol Sci, 11*, 25-33.

West, A. R. & Tseng, K. Y. (2011). Nitric Oxide-Soluble Guanylyl Cyclase-Cyclic GMP Signaling in the Striatum: New Targets for the Treatment of Parkinson's Disease? *Front Syst Neurosci, 5*, 55.

Winek, C. L. & Murphy, K. L. (1984). The rate and kinetic order of ethanol elimination. *Forensic Sci Int, 25*, 159-166.

Wozniak, B., Musialkiewicz, D., Wozniak, A., Drewa, G., Drewa, T., Drewa, S., Mila-Kierzenkowska, C., Porzych, M. & Musialkiewicz, M. (2008). Lack of changes in the concentration of thiobarbituric acid-reactive substances (TBARS). and in the activities of erythrocyte antioxidant enzymes in alcohol-dependent patients after detoxification. *Med Sci Monit 14*, CR32-36.

Xiao, Y., Yan, W., Lu, L., Wang, Y., Lu, W., Cao, Y. & Cai, W. (2015). p38/p53/miR-200a-3p feedback loop promotes oxidative stress-mediated liver cell death. *Cell Cycle*.

Yaldizli, O., Wurst, F. M., Euler, S., Willi, B. & Wiesbeck, G. (2006). Multiple cerebral metastases mimicking Wernicke's encephalopathy in a chronic alcoholic. *Alcohol Alcohol, 41*, 678-680.

Yan, L. J. (2009). Analysis of oxidative modification of proteins. *Curr Protoc Protein Sci*, Chapter *14*, Unit 14 14.

Yan, L. J. (2014). Positive oxidative stress in aging and aging-related disease tolerance. *Redox Biol*, *2***C,** 165-169.

Yan, L. J., Christians, E. S., Liu, L., Xiao, X., Sohal, R. S. & Benjamin, I. J. (2002). Mouse heat shock transcription factor 1 deficiency alters cardiac redox homeostasis and increases mitochondrial oxidative damage. *EMBO. J 21*, 5164-5172.

Yi, K. D., Covey, D. F. & Simpkins, J. W. (2009). Mechanism of okadaic acid-induced neuronal death and the effect of estrogens. *J Neurochem*, *108*, 732-740.

Yuksel, N., Uzbay, I. T., Karakilic, H., Aki, O. E., Etik, C. & Erbas, D. (2005). Increased serum nitrite/nitrate (NOx) and malondialdehyde (MDA) levels during alcohol withdrawal in alcoholic patients. *Pharmacopsychiatry*, *38*, 95-96.

Zaulyanov, L. L., Green, P. S. & Simpkins, J. W. (1999). Glutamate receptor requirement for neuronal death from anoxia-reoxygenation: an in Vitro model for assessment of the neuroprotective effects of estrogens. *Cell Mol Neurobiol*, *19*, 705-718.

Zhou, Z., Wang, L., Song, Z., Saari, J. T., McClain, C. J. & Kang Y. J. (2005). Zinc supplementation prevents alcoholic liver injury in mice through attenuation of oxidative stress. *Am J Pathol*, *166*, 1681-1690.

In: Drug Overdoses and Alcohol Withdrawal   ISBN: 978-1-63483-873-3
Editor: David P. Morales   © 2016 Nova Science Publishers, Inc.

Chapter 4

ALCOHOL WITHDRAWAL: PREVALENCE, TRENDS AND MANAGEMENT

Nadene Fair and Joyce Akwe
Atlanta VA Medical Center, Emory
University School of Medicine, Atlanta GA, US
Morehouse School of Medicine, Atlanta, GA, US

ABSTRACT

Alcohol Use Disorder and its myriad of complications are frequently encountered by Physicians each year. In the United States, it is estimated that approximately 8 million individuals suffer with Alcohol Use Disorder and approximately five hundred thousand will have symptoms of withdrawal, warranting some form of pharmacologic treatment each year. In individuals who are long-term alcohol consumers, reducing or stopping alcohol use suddenly leads to Alcohol Withdrawal Syndromes (AWS), a well-defined cluster of symptoms that range from mild tremors to withdrawal seizures and delirium tremens. In the United States, the estimated healthcare costs due to alcohol withdrawal, in 1998 was close to one hundred and eighty five billion dollars. Some of the costs of alcohol abuse such as domestic violence, child abuse, or loss of a future earnings and health were not even included in these estimates. Additionally, the morbidity and mortality associated with alcohol withdrawal makes it a topic of great importance. It is essential for physicians to be able to identify patients at risk of going into withdrawal and appropriately prevent, and manage all aspects of alcohol withdrawal so as to avoid the associated morbidity, mortality and costly hospital admissions.

This chapter will discuss the epidemiology of alcohol withdrawal, the pathophysiology, the diagnostic criteria for the various manifestations of alcohol withdrawal and the management. There are areas of controversy that exist in the clinical management of Alcohol withdrawal-where to treat and when and how to use medication-these will also be discussed. Recent findings and new treatment options will be reviewed.

INTRODUCTION

Alcohol withdrawal syndromes is a spectrum of symptoms that start manifesting a few hours after the last drink of alcohol and may last up to a week from the last drink. Alcohol is the most commonly abused substances in the United States of America, and so it is no surprise that there is a high incidence of alcohol withdrawal syndromes in the United States of America. Based on the 2013 National Survey on Drug Use and Health, 52.2 percent of Americans aged 12 or older were alcohol drinkers. This percentage translated to estimate 136.9 million alcohol drinkers in 2013 [1]. Approximately 8 million individuals suffer with alcohol withdrawal syndromes; and approximately five hundred will have symptoms of withdrawal, warranting some form of pharmacologic treatment each year [2].

Alcohol withdrawal syndrome results from sudden reduction in chronic alcohol use. Excessive alcohol drinking for even one week can lead to mild withdrawal symptoms, and excessive drinking for over one month leads to significant withdrawal symptoms [4].

PATHOPHYSIOLOGY

The effects of alcohol are due to the direct action of alcohol on both the main inhibitory and excitatory neurotransmission systems. The brain maintains its neurochemical balance through inhibitory and excitatory neurotramissions.

Alcohol is a main central nervous system depressant. It enhances the inhibitory tone and inhibits the excitatory tone.

Alcohol directly enhances the transmission of gamma-aminobutyric acid (GABA) which is a major inhibitory neurotransmitter in the brain. GABA acts through the GABA-A receptors with a resulting neuronal inhibition.

The GABA receptor complex has specific binding sites for alcohol [3], so the transmission of GABA is directly enhanced by alcohol. Inhibition in the neuronal activity causes the sedative effects of alcohol. These inhibitory effects also lead to motor incoordination and cognitive impairment, which are commonly encountered in alcoholics. On the other hand, alcohol inhibits glutamate induced excitation [4, 5]. Glutamate is one of the major excitatory amino acids in the brain. Glutamate binds to NMDA (N-methyl-D-aspartate) receptors causing calcium influx which leads to neuronal excitation.

Cessation or a reduction in chronic alcohol levels causes a decrease in the inhibitory tone and an unregulated excess excitation. These two processes lead to the array of clinical symptoms of alcohol withdrawal syndrome.

The duration of alcohol consumption has been shown to directly correlate to the severity of alcohol withdrawal [6]. Some people have a genetic predisposition to having more severe alcohol withdrawal symptoms than others.

Diagnostic Criteria for Alcohol Withdrawal

Alcohol withdrawal symptoms occur in people who stop drinking for hours to days after they have been drinking for long periods of time.

Minor or early withdrawal symptoms start 6-36 hours after the last drink. Minor withdrawal symptoms include: tremors, anxiety, diaphoresis, palpitations, loss of appetite, nausea, and or vomiting. Patients experiencing minor withdrawal symptoms are usually in their normal mental status. These early symptoms may progress to more severe symptoms if left untreated. Minor symptoms resolve within 1-2 days.

Alcohol withdrawal seizures usually occur 6-48 hours from the last drink. There have been some reports of seizures just 2 hours post alcohol consumption [7]. Seizures due to alcohol withdrawal are usually single episodes or short, brief gusts of generalized tonic-clonic seizures with short post ictal periods. Seizures are more common in people who have been drinking steadily for many years [8]. Status epilepticus are rare.

Alcoholic hallucinations would occur 12 to 48 hours post drinking and resolve with 1-2 days. These are different from Delirium tremens which occur later and may last for up to a week. Alcohol hallucinations are usually visual, but auditory and/or tactile hallucinations are not uncommon. These patients are orientated and have normal vital signs [9]. Alcohol hallucinations have been associated with decreased thiamine levels [10] and genetics [11].

Delirium tremens usually start 48-96 hours after the last drink and may last for up to a week. Delirium tremens is characterized by hallucinations, fevers, disorientation, diaphoresis, agitation, tachycardia, hypertension and delirium. Delirium is the only symptom which is always present. The manifestations of the autonomic hyperactivity may vary.

Patients suffering from Delirium tremens may present with respiratory alkalosis with a very high PH [12] because alcohol is a respiratory depressant with resulting rebound hyperventilation.

Risk Factors for Withdrawals

The intensity of withdrawal symptoms usually gets worse with successive episodes of withdrawals [13]. Certain factors have been identified to be associated with delirium tremens. These factors include: a history of sustained drinking, previous episodes of delirium tremens, age greater than 30, alcohol withdrawal symptoms despite elevated blood alcohol levels, multiple co morbidities or concurrent medical conditions and alcohol withdrawal symptoms presenting long after the last drink [14-18].

Management

Morbidity and mortality in alcohol withdrawal syndromes is dependent upon the rapidity with which susceptible patients can be identified and precautions instituted as well as prompt diagnosis and appropriate treatment of the various presentations of alcohol withdrawal.

Goals of Management

The general goals of management, as for all drugs of dependence are instituted by the American Society of Addiction Medicine and are as follows:

1. To provide safe withdrawal and enable the patient to become drug free
2. To provide withdrawal that is humane and protects the patient's dignity
3. To prepare the patient for ongoing treatment of the dependency.

Specifically for alcohol withdrawal, the aim should be to prevent the onset of AWS in those patients who are at high risk. For those who are already manifesting symptoms and signs of AWS, treatment goals should be to reduce the severity of the withdrawal symptoms by providing prompt and adequate treatment, to decrease morbidity and mortality associated with severe AWS (prevent seizures, delirium tremens and death), and to get the patient ready for long term abstinence from alcohol use by providing ongoing treatment after withdrawal.

Differentials Diagnosis for ETOH Withdrawals

In addition to making a rapid diagnosis of AWS, the diagnosis has to be accurate, as the management for AWS may actually worsen other conditions that may present like AWS. The DSM-5 criteria for AWS is noted in Table …

DSM-V CRITERIA FOR ALCOHOL WITHDRAWAL SYNDROME
A. Cessation or reduction in alcohol intake, which has been prolonged and heavy.

B. A plus any two of the following symptoms developing within several hours to a few days:
  Autonomic Hyperactivity Insomnia Worsening tremor
  Vomiting and Nausea Anxiety
 Hallucinations-visual/tactile/auditory
  Psychomotor Agitation Grand-mal Seizures

C. The symptoms from B cause clinically significant distress or impairment in social, occupational or other important areas of functioning.
D. The above symptoms are not due to general medical conditions and are not better accounted for by another mental disorder, intoxication or withdrawal from other sedatives.

AWS has a spectrum of presentations as noted above. These presentations range from minor nonspecific symptoms to severe life threatening symptoms such as those associated with delirium tremens. As such there are several medical and psychiatric conditions that may present like AWS. These include but are not limited to those listed in the Table below.

DIFFERENTIAL DIAGNOSIS FOR ALCOHOL WITHDRAWAL	
Thyrotoxicosis	Addison Disease
Status Epiliecpticus	Pancreatitis
Hypoglycemia	Hypophosphatemia
Hypomagnesemia	Bipolar Affective Disorder
Panic Disorder	Depression
Insomnia	Dysthymic disorder
Drug Toxicities	Wernicke Encephalopathy
Drug Withdrawals	Social Phobia
CNS infection or bleed	Alcoholic Ketoacidosis

The history and physical examination establishes the diagnosis and severity of AWS: Table ... highlights some key points to determine during the assessment,

HISTORY, PHYSICAL EXAMINATION AND WORKUP OF PATIENT WITH ALCOHOL WITHDRAWAL SYNDROME		
HISTORY	PHYSICAL EXAMINATION[#]	BASIC WORK UP
Length of alcohol use	Temperature/Pulse/BP	Complete blood count
When was the last drink	Arrhythmias	Complete metabolic panel
How much alcohol was taken	Heart failure	Urine drug screen
Any prior alcohol withdrawal symptoms +	Pancreatitis	Magnesium
Other drugs abused-street/prescription	Liver disease	Phosphorus
Coexisting Medical/Psychiatric conditions	GIBleed	Blood alcohol level
Symptoms being experienced[*]	Coronary Artery Disease	EKG
All medications-OTC/prescribed-certain medications can blunt the manifestations of AWS	Infections	
	CNS impairment	

[*]Symptoms to note can be related to time after stopping alcohol and help in determining the severity of the withdrawal.
[#]Looking for signs of AWS and of associated disorders + Kindling-the intensity of withdrawal symptoms increase with successive episodes of withdrawal.

Symptoms and timeline were discussed above. The table below summarizes this information.

SYMPTOMS AND TIMELINE IN ALCOHOL WITHDRAWAL SYNDROME	
SYMPTOMS	TIME OF APPEARANCE AFTER STOPPING ALCOHOL
Minor: insomnia, tremors, GI upset, mild anxiety Anorexia, palpitations, headache, diaphoresis	6-12 hours
Hallucinations-visual, tactile, auditory	12-24 hours
Seizures-generalized tonic - clonic	24-48 hours-seizures may however occur as early as 2 hours after cessation of alcohol
Delirium Tremens-hallucinations, disorientation, tachycardia, diaphoresis, agitation, hypotension, low grade temperature.	48-72 hours with symptoms peaking at 5 days after stopping

The severity of alcohol withdrawal can be broadly divided into three stages. There are two main scales that are used for the assessment and management of AWS, The Clinical Institute Withdrawal Assessment for Alcohol (CIWA) for inpatient and the Short Alcohol Withdrawal Scale (SAWS) for outpatient. Both have limitations but are still being used in most facilities. There are of course other AW scoring methods - the Modified severity assessment scale and the Minnesota Detoxification Scale.

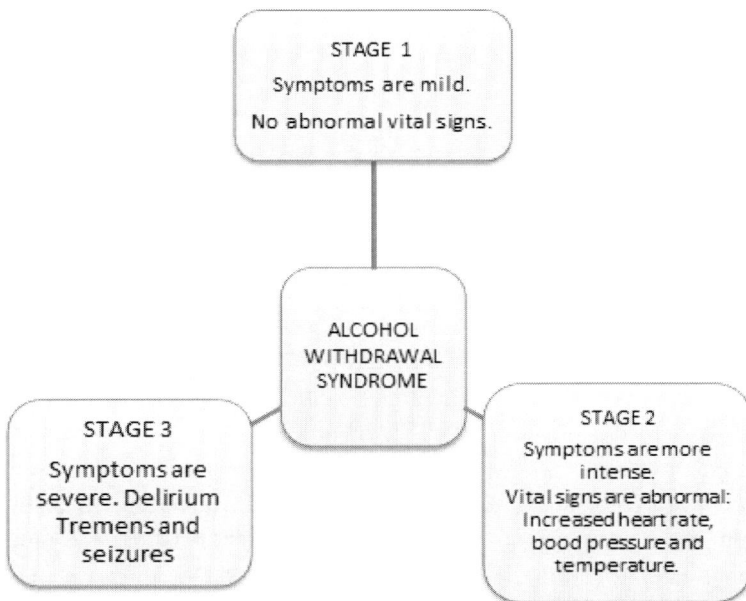

STAGE 1
Symptoms are mild.
No abnormal vital signs.

ALCOHOL WITHDRAWAL SYNDROME

STAGE 3
Symptoms are severe. Delirium Tremens and seizures

STAGE 2
Symptoms are more intense.
Vital signs are abnormal:
Increased heart rate, bood pressure and temperature.

Triage

The choice of treatment setting also impacts the outcome in the management of AWS. The physician must be able to determine the level of care that the patient will require to safely and effectively undergo withdrawal.

Patients with AWS may be cared for in an ambulatory setting as well as inpatient setting. For patients who are being admitted to a facility, the physician then has to determine the level of care-floor admission vs ICU. It is also important to determine on a day to day basis if there is a need to escalate the level of care given due to complications of the withdrawal process or the treatment being given for AWS.

Inpatient vs Ambulatory Management (When to Admit and When to Consider Out-Patient Detox)

There are no specific criteria to determine in where the patient with AWS is to be treated. Generally speaking patients may be treated in an out-patient setting if they are willing to participate in an outpatient program and have access to and from the program on a daily basis and or as specified by the physician. Patients should have a sober person supporting them during this process, preferable an individual who can hold the patient accountable and recognize any adverse event that may be occurring during the process. Ideally, patients with AWS undergoing outpatient detox should have no medical or psychiatric conditions that would complicate the process. If certain chronic medical conditions are well controlled some patients may undergo outpatient detox. Additionally patients should have no other substance abuse issues, should not be cognitively impaired and should have no suicidal ideation or features of psychosis. The CIWA score should ideally be less than 15 with no prior history of alcohol withdrawal seizures or Delirium Tremens. Of course, patients should be able to take oral medications. Patients are required to have daily assessments and to take medications on a fixed schedule. They are usually given a small amount of the medications at each visit. Patients with AWS are not eligible for outpatient treatment if they have abnormal laboratory findings, have poorly controlled chronic medical conditions such as diabetes mellitus, congestive heart failure or COPD or if they have any acute illnesses.

Table ... summarizes the main factors to consider when determining if a patient with AWS is an appropriate candidate for outpatient therapy. Of note if a patient is at risk for seizures and DTs and the physician still determines that outpatient detoxification is possible, the patient should undergo a longer treatment period - 2 weeks as opposed to 5 days.

FACTORS THAT HELP DETERMINE IF PATIENT WITH AWS QUALIFIES FOR OUTPATIENT CARE
Mild to moderate symptoms of AW present-stages 1-2 CIWA < 15

- The patient wants to be detoxified and is willing to participate in outpatient care
- The patient has a sober support individual
- The patient should have daily access to transportation to and from the outpatient clinic: patient cannot drive self
- The patient should have the ability to take medications by mouth.
- There should be no other substance abuse problems
- There should be no psychotic or suicidal features present in the patient
- The patient must not be cognitively impaired.
- There should be no prior history of alcohol withdrawal seizures or delirium tremens
- Chronic medical illnesses should be absent or well controlled

Inpatient Triage-Choice of Disposition (Floor, ICU, Etc.)

Patients with AWS are usually admitted for detoxification if they do not meet the requirements for outpatient care. These are usually patients with severe AW symptoms-AW seizures, Delirium Tremens, a past history of prior AW seizures and or DTs and multiple past detoxification attempts. Patients with concomitant medical and psychiatric conditions such as suicidal ideation are usually admitted for closer monitoring especially if they have recently consumed a lot of alcohol and have no reliable support network to assist them during the withdrawal process. Pregnant patients are all admitted for detox. Most patients may be appropriately and effectively managed on a floor unit with telemetry monitoring and close observation. However patients diagnosed with AWS who are undergoing the following symptoms should be triaged to a higher level of care:

Acute confusion	Hallucinations
Severe tremor	Autonomic disturbances
Confusion	Ataxia
Nystagmus	Hypotension
Ocular palsies	Hypothermia

Features of Wernicke

Table ... shows the things to look for in a patient with AWS that would determine place them in the ICU.

It is ultimately left up to the physician to determine based on the patients history and physical examination the best environment for care.

FACTORS TO HELP DETERMINE WHICH PATIENTS WITH AWS MAY NEED ICU ADMISSION
• Cardiac disease-heart failure/arrhythmias, angina, recent MI
• Renal disease-renal insufficiency, marked acid-base disturbances, severe electrolyte abnormalities
• Respiratory insufficiency-hypoxemia/hypercarbia/pneumonia/copd/ hypocarbia/asthma
• Potentially serious infections-wounds/pneumonia/trauma/UTI
• GI pathology-pancreatitis/hepatic insufficiency/GI bleed
• Persistent hyperthermia
• Rhabdomyolysis
• The need for high doses of sedatives/frequent doses of medication/IV infusion to control symptoms
• A history of prior AW complications
• Age >40

MANAGEMENT

In general, the care of patients with AWS comprises non-pharmacologic and pharmacologic care. Patients with AWS undergoing detox should be ideally kept in a quiet well lit room with limited contact with people. However they should be re oriented periodically and an easily visible calendar or clock should be placed in the room. Special attention should be paid to their fluid balance and nutrition ensuring that they do not become dehydrated or malnourished during the detoxification process. Reassurance and encouragement as well as mental health care also form a basis of general care (see Table … below). It is prudent to monitor patients with AWS closely for complications and prevent or rapidly correct any such events. Patients with severe AWS may become dehydrated through vomiting, diaphoresis, fever, agitation, increased metabolic rate and or hyperthermia. Dehydration in the setting of AWS leads to increased autonomic dysfunction and hypotension making the treatment of AWS more difficult. Always check for decompensated cardiac/liver function when calculating how much fluid to give. Patients may be treated with normal saline at first and then 5% dextrose can be given after the patient is hemodynamically stable and or thiamine is given. Electrolytes should be monitored and repleted when necessary, especially magnesium - as hypomagnesemia reduces seizure threshold, reduces thiamine absorption and may make the repletion of potassium difficult. Complications from alcohol use may also manifest or worsen during the withdrawal period-liver failure/pancreatitis/sub arachnoid or sub-dural hematoma or GI Bleed. Physicians should be on the look-out for delirium secondary to infectious processes or head injury, as well as hypoglycemia. Always give IV thiamine before giving IV glucose to these patients. Since these patients are usually not eating, they may manifest starvation ketosis in addition to alcoholic ketoacidosis with elevated levels of beta hydroxyl butyrate and decreased PH. IV thiamine then D5S and KCL IV can be used to treat starvation ketosis.

GENERAL CARE OF THE PATIENT WITH AWS
• Quiet environment
• Precautions-fall/aspiration/seizure
• Well lit surroundings
• Limited interpersonal interaction
• Frequent reorientation
• Correct abnormalities in fluid balance
• Correct electrolyte abnormalities
• Nutritional support-MVI, thiamine
• Prevent/treat complications

MEDICATION CHOICES

Medication use in patients with AWS is to prevent/treat symptoms. Control of agitation is key in the management of these patients. Ideally, parenteral rapid-acting sedative agents that are cross tolerant with alcohol and produce light somnolence are the drugs of choice. Physicians are still in disagreement with which medications are the best to use and the best prescribing schedule: symptomatic treatment-that is symptom triggered dosing versus fixed schedule dosing with long acting benzodiazepines.

Symptom triggered dosing uses smaller doses of medications, fewer side effects (less sedation and respiratory depression) and shorter hospital stay. There have been several studies done looking at different pharmacologic therapies that can be used in the treatment of AWS and over the years, barbituates, phenothiazines, alcohol itself and carbamazepine has been used and studied. Sedative hypnotic drugs are a grade A recommendation - in the treatment of AWS - with benzodiazepines being the treatment of choice. Benzodiazepines have been proven to the safest and most effective medications to date. Benzodiazepines prevent and alleviate withdrawal symptoms and also decrease the occurrence of seizures and delirium tremens. Summarily, shorter acting benzodiazepines are safer in the elderly and patients with liver disease and can be administered in the symptom-triggered validated protocols such as the CIWA. While longer acting benzodiazepines are least expensive, the most studied, are more effective in preventing seizures and provide a smoother withdrawal process. Fixed schedule dosing of benzodiazepines regardless of whether the patient has symptoms means that patients will not need frequent observation for symptom assessment. Fixed schedule dosing may also be used in patients with AWS in which their comorbid medical illnesses or post-operative status makes it difficult to assess their withdrawal symptoms. In facilities where there is a high patient to clinician ration this sort of treatment is necessary. Other medications such as, clonidine, beta blockers and carbamazepine treat some but not all symptoms in AWS and are usually used along with benzodiazepines.

BENZODIAZEPINES

The benzodiazepines have been studied extensively with several meta-analyses showing that it is the best first line drug to use for all stages of AWS. It is primarily used to treat the psychomotor agitation that occurs in AWS and has been shown to prevent the worsening of AWS, from stage 1 through to stages 2/3. They have been shown to prevent first seizures and secondary seizures in AWS. Benzodiazepines are the medication of choice for the prevention and treatment of DT.

How Do Benzodiazepines Work in AWS?

Benzodiazepines act on the GABA receptors, modulating/stimulating the receptors so that the affinity for the GABA neurotransmitter in increased. This increased attraction of the receptors, results in an increase in the binding of the GABA neurotransmitter leading to more chloride ions crossing the terminal membrane leading to an inhibition in neuronal activity and thus a relative sedation.

Choosing a Benzodiazepine

There are no studies that demonstrate the efficacy of one benzodiazepine when compared to another. There are several factors to consider when choosing a benzodiazepine in the setting of AWS. The aim of therapy is to cause the production of GABA at a rate that is equivalent to the quantity produced by alcohol thus counteracting the psychomotor agitation. Some of the factors considered in order to achieve the desired goal include:

#Onset of action:
   #Duration of action
   #Route of Administration
   #Patients Hepatic function
   #Clinic or Hospital Formulary
#Duration of Action:

Long-acting-Diazepam (Valium), Chlordiazepoxide (Librium) - see Table … for recommended dosing-these are the most commonly used long acting benzodiazepines used for the treatment of AWS. These benzodiazepines are oxidized to form active metabolites that have long half-lives, so there is a smoother decline in the plasma level of the drug leading to a prolongation of the sedative and anxiolytic effects and hence less of a chance of break through or rebound symptoms. In patients with liver disease and the elderly, there will be unpredictable metabolism of these long acting benzos thus causing over sedation. Diazepam in particular is very lipophilic and so is rapidly distributed in the CNS causing a rapid onset of action.

Unfortunately this process is also rapidly reversed when the diazepam then redistributes in the peripheral fat stores, in an unpredictable manner again quickly leading to over sedation. These benzodiazepines may be used in the outpatient setting in which case it is recommended that the patient be seen daily, their alcohol level be checked and the medications be dispensed on a daily basis. The medication is usually tapered over 5-7 days. These benzodiazepines should be stopped if the patient relapses.

Short-acting-Lorazepam (Ativan), Oxazepam (Serax) - These benzodiazepines have no active metabolites. Lorazepam undergoes glucuronidation in the liver-a process which is preserved in cirrhotic livers. The inactive metabolite produced is then eliminated. These short-acting agents are preferred when treating AWS in patients with impaired hepatic (advanced cirrhosis/acute alcoholic hepatitis) or and or renal function.

They are also the drug of choice to be used in the elderly. Lorazepam has the distinction of having several routes of admission with similar efficacy-IV/IM and PO. The draw back with these short acting drugs is the rapidity with which patients may develop dependence and subsequently symptomatic withdrawal.

It is important to pay attention to dosing of these medications. The dose of the drug given is dependent on the patient's clinical presentation, the presence of comorbidities, and the patient's risk factor and ability to tolerate DTs. It is interesting to note that the genetic make-up of a patient may contribute to their response to benzodiazepines possibly explaining why in some patients an inordinately high amount of the medication may be needed to achieve the desired sedating effect. There are actually studies that have shown that in DTs, the dose of the benzodiazepine may far exceed that which would be considered normal-massive doses e.g., >2g diazepam/48 hours.

#Route of Administration: In clinically stable patients with mild to moderate symptoms of AW and most outpatient settings, benzodiazepines may be administered orally. In patients with seizures or delirium tremens-IV route is preferred. When patients first present with AWS-tremulousness, the IV route is recommended as it will ensure rapid absorption, rapid onset and thus prevent symptoms from progressing. It is usually recommended to avoid IM injections unless absolutely necessary, because the absorption of the drug will be unpredictable.

Overall symptom triggered therapy is considered the best way to administer these medications as it will lead to the use of less medication, resulting in less SE/sedation and less cost.

It is used in conjunction with the clinical Institute Withdrawal Assessment for Alcohol Scale or some equivalent scale to determine the need for sedation. Evaluations are frequent initially 10-15 minute intervals in patients with severe presentation and increased to hourly intervals once the patients severe symptoms are controlled. As the patient gets more stable, the interval of assessment can be increased. This is of course time consuming, subject to administrator error and is labor intensive but it is offset by the above mentioned advantages.

In heavily sedated patients or intubated patients the CIWAS-Ar cannot be suitable administered, the recommendation is that the RASS scale-Richmond Agitation Sedation Scale-see Table … be used to determine the need for benzodiazepines. Fixed schedule therapy with these drugs does not have a lot of evidence to support it and it is usually used in situations where staffing for frequent assessment is limited.

ANTICONVULSANTS

Anticonvulsants are another group of drugs that have been studied in the treatment of AWS and have been shown to actually help. They are not as effective as benzodiazepines.

Carbamazepine is the most studied drug in this class. It has been shown to be safe and effective. It is mostly used in the outpatient setting and in the treatment of mild AWS. It does not potentiate alcohol intoxication, is less sedative and does not result in abuse. It has been shown to decrease anxiety symptoms and prevent post treatment relapses. There is however no evidence to support its use in the treatment of DTs. It should not be used to treat isolated seizures caused from AW as the majority of seizures from withdrawal are self-limiting. Side effects of carbamazepine include dizziness, nausea, vomiting, ataxia, and diplopia.

Other anticonvulsants have limited data to support us in the treatment of AWS. Of note Lamotrigine and Topiramate decrease AW severity and decreases the amount of benzodiazepines that need to be given.

Phenytoin is not effective in the treatment of AW.

OTHER MEDICATIONS

Other medications can be used to help reduce the intensity and frequency of AWS and also to help reduce the dosage of BZD used in the treatment. However there are not many studies available and they may mask the symptoms in AWS that are used to assess severity.

Baclofen: A selective GABA B receptor agonist.

Decreases the severity of withdrawal symptoms and prevents post treatment relapses. It has not been shown to be effective in controlling severe symptoms so should not be used for the treatment of acute severe alcohol withdrawal.

Beta-blockers: This is adjunctive medications may be given with benzodiazepines to help reduce persistent agitation. They can mask changes in the heart rate or blood pressure and thus cause an inaccurate assessment of symptoms in AWS. Beta blockers have not been shown to prevent the development of seizures or DTs. Additionally beta blockers have been shown to cause delirium.

Beta blockers should not be used for the treatment of acute severe alcohol withdrawal. Patients who are already on beta blockers should be maintained on them.

Alpha-2 agonists: This medication can also be used as adjunct therapy to reduce some of the withdrawal symptoms. There are currently no studies to show that they prevent the development of seizures or DTs and as such are not used in the primary treatment of acute severe AWS.

Antipsychotics: These medications lower the seizure threshold and it is not recommended that they be used routinely in patients with AWS. The most commonly used antipsychotic is haloperidol which can be used to control anxiousness, hallucinations and combativeness. It is used only in conjunction with BZD, when the BZD therapy is not controlling the patient's symptoms. The patient should be on telemetry while receiving this medication.

Phenobarbital: Phenobarbital also acts on the GABA-A receptors in the central nervous system increasing the affinity of the GABA binding to its receptors leading to an increase in the inhibitory effect. This inhibition counteracts the excitatory surge during DTs. The drawback to the use of phenobarbital is that it has a long half-life that causes it to be difficult to titrate to a dose that is effective in sedating the patient while allowing for the patient to wake up. Additionally, phenobarbital has a higher level or associated respiratory depression and coma compared to BZD.

Propofol: Propofol is thought to modify the GABA-A and NDMA receptors. In the ICU setting, it allows for rapid onset of sedation and when stopped allows for the patient to be awaken suddenly. Its short half-life makes it titratable. Propofol does however require intense monitoring and can cause hypotension and bradycardia. Side effects include pancreatitis secondary to increased lipid load as it is a lipid emulsion and this can complicate the picture in a patient already undergoing AWS.

Thiamine and Folic acid: Thiamine lowers the risk of Wernicke encephalopathy.

Ethanol: There are very few studies to support the use of ethanol in the treatment of AWS. It was used in the past IV or PO to prevent or treat AWS. The efficacy, the optimal way to give ethanol and what complications to expect are not well defined and as such it makes ethanol a controversial alternative medication. Additionally the toxicities associated with ethanol (pancreatitis, hepatitis, bone marrow suppression and narrow therapeutic index) makes ethanol a poor drug of choice in the setting of AWS.

Sodium Oxybate: This is a sodium salt of gamma hydroxybutyric acid (GHB).

GHB is structurally similar to GABA and may indirectly activate the GAB-A receptors, thus suppressing the excitatory symptoms of AWS. On the other hand, GHB can also cause symptoms similar to those in AWS because of the release of dopamine in the CNS.

This drug is currently being used in Europe where it has been shown that in treating acute AWS, sodium oxybate decreases the symptoms of withdrawal compared to placebo and with symptoms that are moderate to severe, it acts equally or more effective than diazepam. The side effects of vertigo, drowsiness, diarrhea and gastric upset are commonly reported and are relatively well tolerated. It is still being investigated for use in the US.

Protocols

The most common and validated protocol used in the treatment of AWS is the CIWA-Ar. This protocol is a ten item survey that is used to assess the patient's symptoms and then determines the severity of the symptoms based on the scores obtained. Medication is then given based on this assessment, Point range from 0-67 and the signs and symptoms assessed include sweating/ anxiety/tremors, hallucinations, HA and disorientation or clouding of the senses. This protocol has been shown in various studies to reduce the duration of treatment, decrease ICU admission and avoid the risk of over sedation. It is however staff and time consuming-it takes at least 5-15minutes to conduct a CIWA-Ar assessment and is dependent on staff being properly trained to recognize signs and symptoms of AWS so as to avoid protocol errors.

It is worthwhile noting that fixed dosing does avoid protocol errors but bears the risk for longer hospital stays and over sedation. There are other protocols as mentioned before that are essentially derived from CIWA-Ar and they too have reduced use of benzos and reduced treatment times.

These scales are however dependent on the patient's ability to respond to question and follow commands and so cannot be used in certain patient populations. Additionally, these scales should be used as adjunct to a high clinical suspicion and thorough history, in the diagnosis of AWS as patients with withdrawal symptoms may be mis-diagnosed as having infection, pain or other causes of delirium or patients who are known to have alcohol use disorder may be treated as AWS when an unrelated condition could be causing the symptoms.

DELIRIUM TREMENS

Commonly known as DTs, is the most severe form of AWS. It is thought to occur in about 5% of patients hospitalized for AWS. Patients present with altered mental status and sympathetic overdrive that can culminate in cardiovascular collapse.

It has a high mortality rate and is a medical emergency. As such it needs to be recognized and treated early. DT is usually as a result of under treatment or lack of treatment of early AWS. It typically presents 3-5 days after the last drink. Symptoms include severe agitation, disorientation, tremor, increased ANS symptoms (palpitations, tremor, sweating, hypertension, and tachypnea) and hallucinations.

These symptoms may be present for up to a week. Risk factors include patients with a CiWA-Ar score greater than 15, history of DTs or seizures, the presence of other illnesses (hypokalemia, hypomagnesemia, low platelets and cardiac, GI and respiratory diseases), patients withdrawing while still having high levels of blood alcohol, older age, use of other depressant agents, and patients with more days since last drink. Death in this setting usually occurs from hyperthermia, concomitant medical illnesses, complication of seizures and cardiac arrhythmias.

It is best to prevent DTs. Therefore, early detection and treatment of the early withdrawal symptoms and the identification of risk factors that predispose to DTs. Concomitant medical problems should also be rapidly controlled.

The treatment goals: 1. Control agitation 2. Decrease the risk of seizures.

DTs are best treated in an ICU setting or in a locked inpatient ward.

The work up is aimed at confirming the diagnosis of DTs – ruling out medical conditions that have similar presentations or that can complicate DTs. Blood work such as chemistry-magnesium, pancreatic enzymes, LFT,CBC and BAL. The patient requires supportive care with frequent/continuous vital sign assessment in a quiet well lit room with frequent reorientation to time place and person.

Thiamine should be given so as to prevent Wernicke's encephalopathy. Calculate volume deficits and replete along with any electrolyte deficiencies. Treat agitation, promote sleep and raise the seizure threshold. BZD are the mainstay of treatment of DTs, IV in high enough doses to get the patient to a dozing but easily arousable state. There are many different tapering regimens.

Prognosis

Delirium tremens has been reported in 5-12% of patients suffering from alcohol dependence. If left untreated, mortality rates could be as high as 40%. The mortality rate falls to about 5% with appropriate medical treatment [19]. Deaths from delirium tremens have been attributed to electrolyte abnormalities, cardiovascular complications, head trauma and aspiration.

Alcohol withdrawal seizures have been reported in about 10% of alcohol withdrawal patients. Patients who have been drinking alcohol steadily for several years may have higher percentages of alcohol withdrawal seizures [8].

Prevention

The focus of prevention is on early identification of alcohol use disorder or treatment of early symptoms that could lead to more severe complications. Standardized questionnaires by the United States Task Force [20] should be used as a screening tool for these patients. Patients with alcohol use disorder can benefit from structured intervention to reduce, stop drinking, and stay sober. Once patient develop more severe dependence to alcohol, medical supervision is required for management of withdrawals. Alcohol withdrawal syndrome may complicate recovery after surgery, so patients should be screened during preoperative evaluation. In cases of elective surgery, surgery could be scheduled 7-10 days after the last drink.

REFERENCES

[1]   http://store.samhsa.gov/home.
[2]   Kosten, T. R., O'Connor, P. G. Management of drug and alcohol withdrawal. *N. Engl. J. Med.* 2003; 348:1786.
[3]   Hic, S. J., Ye, Q., Wick, M. J. et al. Sites of alcohol and volatile anaesthetic action on GABA(A) and glycine receptors. *Nature* 1997; 389:385.
[4]   Hoffman, P. L., Grant, K. A., Snell, L. D. et al. NMDA receptors: role in ethanol withdrawal seizures. *Ann. N. Y. Acad. Sci.* 1992; 654:52.
[5]   Tsai, G., Gastfriend, D. R., Coyle, J. T. The glutamatergic basis of human alcoholism. *Am. J. Psychiatry* 1995; 152:332.

[6]   Isbell, H., Fraser, H. F., Wikler, A. et al. An experimental study of the etiology of rum fits and delirium tremens. *Q. J. Stud. Alcohol* 1955; 16: 1.

[7]   Victor, M., Brausch, C. The role of abstinence in the genesis of alcoholic epilepsy. *Epilepsia* 1967; 8:1.

[8]   Victor, M., Adams, R. D. The effect of alcohol on the nervous system. *Res. Publ. Assoc. Res. Nerv. Ment. Dis.* 1953; 32:526.

[9]   Marchal, C. [Alcohol and epilepsy]. *Rev. Prat.* 1999; 49:383.

[10]   Holzbach, E. Thiamine absorption in alcoholic delirium patients. *J. Stud. Alcohol* 1996; 57:581.

[11]   Limosin, F., Loze, J. Y., Boni, C. et al. The A9 allele of the dopamine transporter gene increases the risk of visual hallucinations during alcohol withdrawal in alcohol-dependent women. *Neurosci. Lett.* 2004; 362:91.

[12]   Dobes, M. Disorders of the acid-base equilibrium in delirium tremens. *Cas. Lek. Cesk.* 1993;132:142-5.

[13]   Booth, B. M., Blow, F. C. The kindling hypothesis: further evidence from a US national study of alcoholic men. *Alcohol Alcohol.* 1993; 28: 593.

[14]   Blondell, R. D. Ambulatory detoxification of patients with alcohol dependence. *Am. Fam. Physician* 2005; 71:495.

[15]   Brown, M. E., Anton, R. F., Malcolm, R., Ballenger, J. C. Alcohol detoxification and withdrawal seizures: clinical support for a kindling hypothesis. *Biol. Psychiatry* 1988; 23:507.

[16]   Ferguson, J. A., Suelzer, C. J., Eckert, G. J. et al. Risk factors for delirium tremens development. *J. Gen. Intern. Med.* 1996; 11:410.

[17]   Palmstierna, T. A model for predicting alcohol withdrawal delirium. *Psychiatr. Serv.* 2001; 52:820.

[18]   Ballenger, J. C., Post, R. M. Kindling as a model for alcohol withdrawal syndromes. *Br. J. Psychiatry* 1978; 133:1.

[19]   Yost, D. A. Alcohol withdrawal syndrome. *Am. Fam. Physician* 1996; 54:657.

[20]   http://www.samhsa.gov/data/sites/default/files/NSDUHresultsPDFWHT ML2013/Web/NSDUHresults2013.pdf.

****

Bayard, M., McIntyre, J. et al. Alcohol withdrawal syndrome: *American Family Physician* 2004 vol. 69, number 9 1443-1452.

Boston, L. N. alcohol withdrawal. *Lancet* 1908: 1:18.

Hecksel, K. A., Bostwick, J. M., Jaeger, T. M., Cha, S. S. Inappropriate use of symptom triggered therapy for alcohol withdrawal in the general Hospital. *Mayo clinic Proc.* 2008:83; 274.

Hoffman, R. S. et al. Management of moderate and severe alcohol withdrawal syndromes. *Up to date* 2015.

Minozzi, S., Amato, L., Vecchi, S., Dacoli, M. Anticonvulsants for alcohol withdrawal. *Cochrane DatBASE Syst. Rev.* 2010: CD005064.

McKeon, A., Frye, M. A., Delanty, N. The alcohol withdrawal syndrome. *J. Neurol. Neurosurg. Psychiatry* 2008:79;854-862.

Sullivan, J. T., Sykora, K., Schneiderman, J. et al. Assessment of alcohol withdrawal: the revised clinical institute withdrawal assessment for Alcohol scale (CiWA-Ar). *Br. J. Addict.* 1989: 84:1353.

In: Drug Overdoses and Alcohol Withdrawal   ISBN: 978-1-63483-873-3
Editor: David P. Morales   © 2016 Nova Science Publishers, Inc.

Chapter 5

POLYPHARMACY: A KEY ISSUE OF CONTEMPORARY GERIATRIC MEDICINE

Pavel Weber, Hana Meluzínová and Dana Prudius*

Department of Internal Medicine, Geriatrics and Practical Medicine;
Masaryk University and University Hospital; Brno, Czech Republic

ABSTRACT

Diseases and conditions in the elderly are generally characterized by numerous peculiarities. Diseases often tend to accumulate and potentiate each other. In geriatrics *multi-dimensionality* is typical. The elderly patient as a *bio-psycho-social unit* should be even more understood than those in the younger age group in both etiopathogenesis of diseases as well as in clinical practice. Psychological and social problems always appear simultaneously with somatic complaints, which also need to be handled with the same urgency. This applies for primary somatic diseases which are characteristic for advanced age (strokes, degenerative diseases, tumors, immobilisation). In a similar way this also applies for the so called 'primary' mental disorders (dementia, depression, delirium) or so-called geriatric social syndromes (maladaptive geriatric syndrome; syndrome of mistreatment, neglect syndrome and elder abuse syndrome).

Majority of the clinical doctors consider multi-morbidity as an unpleasant phenomenon associated with the decrease in functional

---

* Corresponding author: Prof. Pavel Weber, MD., Ph.D.; Department of Internal Medicine, Geriatrics and Practical Medicine; Masaryk University and University Hospital; Jihlavská 20; 62500 Brno; Czech Republic. Tel: 00420-5-32232509. E-mail: p.weber @ fnbrno.cz.

capacity, cognitive disorders, and moreover the risk of interactions between diseases themselves and their possible pharmacological therapy. In the elderly (especially late old age) multi-morbidity is the rule rather than the exception. Almost half of the people aged 65 to 69 years have two or more chronic diseases. The group of seniors with multi-morbidity has increased significantly especially in the last decade of life (22%). At the age of ≥ 85 y. there are more than 75% multi-morbid persons.

Pitfalls and negatives of multi-morbidity represent:

- Accelerated decline of the functional capacity
- The higher incidence of symptoms and subjective complaints
- The decline of quality of life
- Increased mortality
- Increased risk of hospitalization
- Increased risk of institutionalization (nursing or residential home, etc.)
- Rising health care costs

There is a lack of evidences for a specific treatment of multi-morbid seniors because they are usually excluded from major clinical trials (RCT = randomized clinical trials). The retrospective analysis of five general medical journals with the highest IF states that 284 of RCT from 1995 to 2010 65% of seniors were excluded for multi-morbidity. According to 11 Cochrane Review RCT assessment the presence of typical four chronic diseases (diabetes, heart failure, COPD, stroke) was less than half of the participants in these studies meeting the entry criteria either of the following chronic diagnoses. Multi-morbid seniors usually do not feature in the RCTs. Clinical guidelines generally do not count at all with multi-morbidity and often do not provide recommendations, which would take account of other simultaneously occurring comorbidities. Polypharmacy often justified and effective in the old age depends primarily on co-existing multi-morbidity. Although the individual diseases are quite correctly indicated and treated according to EBM (evidence-based medicine), quite often the possible impending pharmacological interactions recede into the background. Therefore it can be difficult to reveal it. Polypharmacy is also discussed in the situation when the patient is using only one not strictly necessary medicament. To some extent, this concept tends to lead to the noncoordination and the ineffectivity of therapeutic procedures. Polypharmacy may lead to an exponential increase of the risk of side effects and drug interactions (with 6 or more drugs is the risk particularly high according WHO).

The principles of geriatric prescription at a superficial glance may seem to give the impression that the prescription is similar to the one for younger individuals. The prescription for seniors requires understanding of: a clear indication of the drug; the knowledge of dosing; potential side reactions and drug interactions. In the geriatric prescription it is necessary to take into consideration the changes in cognitive function, decreased manual dexterity and vice versa the rise of the need of social support. The principles of prescription in the elderly comprise both the technical expertise of the prescription of drugs and the knowledge of bio-psycho-social factors enabling to meet all the individual needs of seniors.

The elderly are generally more vulnerable, the therapeutic range is narrowing, the compliance is decreasing, interindividual variability of the drug effect and the risk of drug interactions are increasing. In the elderly, there is a rise of gastric pH, on the other hand the stomach and intestinal motility as well as the blood flow to the gastrointestinal tract are decreasing. Despite all these changes the absorption of most drugs in the old age is not significantly affected.

In the elderly, about ½ patients aged 57-85 y. have ≥ 5 drugs. As the age is increasing, the number of drugs is increasing too. At about ½ of the cases wrong combination of drugs is prescribed (drug-drug) and about 1 in 20 has a high risk drugs combination.

The number of potential *drug interactions* grows exponentially with the number of drugs prescribed. The drug interaction may occur with some foodstuffs (absorption, metabolism). Potential side reactions are responsible for 1/5 of all hospitalizations of patients. It can be predicted that almost 1/3 and the mere reduction of the dose of medicament can be eliminated to 2/3 of them. Inappropriate medication by Beers criteria contributes only to 7% of hospitalizations.

Reduction of excessive polypharmacy is a benefit for the patient's health. It improves the treatment adherence and reduces the cost of medication. Scott directly states that no study has shown that the change (reduction) in polypharmacy decreased morbidity or mortality of seniors, but it led to a decline of potential side reactions (35%), costs decrease, and it also improved the compliance of the leftover medication. *The non-prescription of drugs should become a routine.*

The ideal situation of the geriatric prescription creates 1 prescribing doctor and 1 pharmacy. Each new physician increases the probability of potential side reactions by 29%. According to major studies e-prescribing can reduce inappropriate prescribing by 1-24%. Its effect on polypharmacy remains unclear.

Compliance decreases dramatically after ≥ 6 months of the drug usage. If the disease is symptomatic better adherence to the use of drugs occurs. The regular contact between the patient and the doctor is quite essential for improving and maintaining the adherence of an established therapy. Nothing can replace the 'face to face' visits at the doctor's office.

POSSIBLE CRUCIAL FACTORS OF AGING PROCESS ON DRUG USE IN GERIATRIC MEDICINE

The development of human community leads to increasing hope of longer survival and makes the average life expectancy longer. The amount of the elderly, very old and "oldest-old" ($\geq$ 85 y.) people are relatively and also absolutely increasing [48, 88]. The elderly are extremely heterogeneous group of people. The old age life is not easy and there are many exposures - health problems, loneliness, misunderstandings, loss of advisability, self-sufficiency and autonomy, poverty, age segregation and discrimination (ageism) [47, 109, 120].

If we want to perceive the issue of polypharmacy in relation to geriatric medicine and aging process at all correctly, we must first briefly outline some peculiarities and specifics of the elderly population. Old people have usually tight relation to their miscellaneous medication. Without basic knowledge we cannot look on the issue of polypharmacy in the elderly in a sophisticated way and understand it comprehensively. Therefore, the introduction will outline some of the key issues in geriatric medicine, without which you cannot quite understand this complex issue with such a heterogeneous population, which seniors already are today [6, 45].

The consequence of aging is old and very old age (senescence) as a result of multifactorial processes. Its usual manifestation is due to a combination of involutional changes and symptoms of diseases [71], especially those whose occurrence is age-related (e.g., atherosclerosis). The environment importantly influences and modifies the speed of ageing process and occurrence of diseases [63]. About 25% of this variability is genetically conditional and 75% by epigenetic factors, including the influence of the environment and lifestyle, especially diet and physical activity [48].

Health status in old age is a consequence of many factors, including chronic diseases of ageing and many other prevalent reasons that cannot be defined as classic 'diseases' because they do not rise from a single pathologic cause [78]. Many of the signs affecting old people should be considered as independent geriatric giants or syndromes (GS), that are a collection of signs and symptoms with a huge number of potential causes [46, 54, 89].

The *crux of geriatric medicine* is involutionarity caused *decline of health potential, frailty* and *related geriatric syndromes* and *function deficiency* with their multicausal sources.

Geriatric giants [61, 113, 119] represent:

- *immobility* (decubitus, etc.),
- *instability* (vertigo, posture and gait disorders, falls),
- *incontinence,*
- *intellectual disorders* (delirium, dementia and depression),
- *iatrogenia* (dangerous polypharmacy).

As further geriatric syndromes we perceive [8, 92]:

- syndrome of hypomobility, decondition and sarcopenia
- anorexia syndrome and malnutrition
- syndrome of dual combined sensoric deficiency (visual and hearing)
- syndrome of dehydration with subsequent manifestation of acute renal failure
- syndrome of thermoregulatory disturbance
- syndrome of elder abuse, neglect and self-neglect syndrome
- syndrome of geriatric maladaptation
- syndrome of terminal geriatric deterioration - FTT ('failure to thrive')

The above mentioned GS do not always threaten patient's life but they basically influence its quality [25]. Seniors become gradually and completely dependent on other people´s assistance (family, friends, community services, institutional care) [117].

Frailty [35, 95] belongs to key characteristics of especially very old geriatric patients. Frailty is a biologic syndrome of decreased reserves in multiple systems that arise from dysregulation that can develop with ageing and is started by physiological changes of ageing, disease, and/or a lack of activity [35, 81]. These factors play a crucial role in its development and are caused by the diminution of proteosynthesis in the muscles, decline of immune function, growth of the mass of inner fat and reduction of the amount of the share of body water and of the bone mineral density, loss of the whole body mass and muscle strength.

MULTI-MORBIDITY IN OLD AGE: A RISK FACTOR FOR POLYPHARMACY

Multi-morbidity, polymorbidity, polypathy, coprevalence, a phenomenon quite typical for old age, i.e., contemporary existence of many diseases in one individual without either reason or other diseases are causally conditioning [1, 96, 111]. Boyd [12] defines multi-morbidity as the coexistence of two or more chronic diseases, where none can be defined as central to the others. With increasing age, the share of multi-morbidity grows very significantly [62, 73]. In old age it has an essential influence on the clinical picture of diseases, their therapy and prognosis. Consequently to that, there is a diminution in functional capacity of organ systems and disability appears gradually. This in turn leads to restrictions of self-sufficiency and the development of dependence [73].

The interaction between old age and illness causes specific changes in clinical picture of diseases in the elderly [13, 26].

Particularities of illness in old age include:

- Multi-morbidity - parallel occurrence of more illnesses in one person with or without causality relationship
- Mutual causality of social and health situation - each of the changes of the health state in old age influences their social status and vice versa
- Among the specialties of clinical picture of illnesses in old age we can list:

1. *microsymptomathology* - minimal symptoms of diseases (the iceberg phenomenon)
2. *mono- or oligosyptomatology* - sporadic symptoms from those, which occur usually in middle or young age
3. *distant signs* - to the forefront of clinical picture there are symptoms, which belong to the difficulties of other organ than the basic one ("the innocent organ complains, not the sick one")
4. *tendency to chronicity* - even in the diseases which are in younger and middle age acute, moreover in old age there is higher risk of death
5. *tendency to complications* - either of type of "chain reaction" or it is the complication, which does not have the direct relation ("crowd-out effect")

6. *atypical picture* of the diseases - *'For the diseases in the old age it is typical that their running is atypical'*

The proper symptomatology of the crucial disease is usually inconspicuous [102]. In the clinical picture outbalance non-specific and universal symptoms from the secondary brain decompensation. The universal non-specific neurologic and psychiatric symptomatology caused by hypoperfusion (hypoxia) of the brain (transitory ischemic attack-TIA, delirium etc.) belong. The senior's brain is generally affected with the degenerative or vascular changes which can augment the problem. Central nervous system (brain) reacts usually as the first organ [53].

Among the causes of the morbidity in old age the front position [32] is being taken by the diseases of the cardiovascular system conditioned mainly with atherosclerosis [74]. After the age of 60 there is a continuous growth of cardiovascular diseases, such as the coronary heart disease (CHD), stroke, hypertension [24, 121].

For the quality of the senior's life and keeping of self-sufficiency cornerstone is not the presence of the disease itself (or more diseases) but the keeping of self-sufficiency, grade of the disability and development of dependency [10]. The full self-sufficiency can be unchanged even sometimes when there are more diseases present together [1, 76].

The inclination of older population to the occurrence of diseases is higher [78] and the balance of the organ homeostasis is very frail and develops *homeostenosis*. Similar situation we observe in the case of 'primary' mental disorders (dementia, depression, delirium) or in the primary geriatric social syndromes (neglect syndrome, elder abuse, geriatric maladaptation syndrome) - [109]. The stressor is as a rule in psychosocial domain and its clinical manifestation seems most frequently in the cardiovascular sphere (heart failure, angina pectoris, myocard infarct, stroke or venous trombembolism) [3, 105].

The mentioned problems from the somatic, psychic and social sphere which are in the mutual interaction are with difficulty treatable, they are in nature chronic and progressive and they have relatively unfavourable prognosis. They produce a lot of not easily solvable situations and problems to the ill, the relatives and caring facilities [11]. By the 'old old' people (≥ 80 years) the diseases continue in the way, which differ from the progression of the diseases in middle age and they need the different approach which can improve sometimes the health status or at least maintain the self-sufficiency and they prefer the ability go home from the facility of institutional care [80].

The most of the biological functions achieve the top before the 30th year of the life. Some of them fall slightly afterwards linearly. For the everyday activity this decrease has not any practical importance, but can be obvious in the time of bigger stress or in the load (serious disease, trauma, operation etc.). Physiologically diminish hand to hand as the age grows: renal perfusion, the clearance of the creatinin, the maximum heart rate and pulse volume in stress, glucose tolerance, vital capacity of the lungs, body weight cell immunity. On the contrary the total lung capacity and the liver function do not change basically with increasing age. The secretion of the ADH is even growing.

This diminution in physiological reserve capacity does not influence the everyday life but it can influence the ability to recover from the severe disease (serious infection, life threatening internal diseases, operations, traumas etc.) - [94, 105].

Some of the physiological changes can even imitate a disease even if they are just an ordinary component of the ageing. Diabetes mellitus can appear and disappear in the old age. The ability of the insulin to stimulate the take up of the glucose decreases with the age [101, 106]. In the stress or overload situations diabetes can be detected in seniors, but it can disappear when the relations get normal. This situation we can catch and observe often by usage the drugs with diabetiogenic effect by contemporary present polypharmacy from different causes of therapy [34, 43].

The age conditioned metabolic changes, which make the elderly people more vulnerable in their everyday life, are usually mild, but can also importantly influence the development of impaired glucose tolerance [55].

The half of the people 65 years and older have two or more diseases and these can essentially elevate a risk of unfavourable consequences like mortality [103]. In some of the elderly people the cognitive disorder can mimic signs of a severe disease. The therapy of one disease can act in an undesirable way on the other place. Certain combinations of the diseases can elevate the risk of disability and dependency synergistically. The arthrosis as not- live endangering in coexistence with the coronary heart disease co-exist in 1/5 of the elderly, even though the risks of progress of disability are 3- or 4- times higher with one of them alone, the risk of both together is 14-times higher [88].

On the onset and the development of the critical conditions in the elderly following factors can significantly participate: the poor mobility, loneliness, bad eating habits, insufficient hydration, mental deterioration, disturbance of the sight and hearing [47]. The mentioned ill individuals have, as it is with multi-morbidity in old age common, an atypical picture, or they can be without symptoms or the problems are moved to the other organ system. The important role is played also often by rich pharmacotherapy (polypharmacy, contingently excessive polypharmacy) in old age, which can itself cause different organ symptoms (also by the mutual interactions).

PARTICULARITIES IN CHANGES OF FUNCTIONING OF ORGAN SYSTEMS IN OLD AGE

The important alteration in the body composition include the decline of lean body mass (primarily the loss of the muscles) connected with the proportional increase of the inner fat [90, 118]. These basic changeovers are essential determinants of the physiological functions and therapeutic limitations in the old age. For example the diminished muscle tissue is responsible to a certain extent for the decrease of consumption of oxygen during the exercise or overload ($VO_{2max.}$) detectable with the increasing age. Moreover the growth of the body fat increases the distributional volume of lipophile drugs and thus prolongs their pharmacological action. The changes in the body composition in elderly people are probably caused both by the ageing process and different external factors like low physical activity and changed way of catering and pertinent malnourishment. The age changeovers include homeostatic control of disturbed baro-reflex sensitivity, which alone predispose to orthostatic hypotension a worse thermoregulation, which increases the tendency to thermoregulatory disorders (hypothermia) and stroke.

For the doctors there could be sometimes dangerous to be guided by the presumptions, schemes and experience created in younger and middle age patients. The threatening mistake and especially the delay may be serious especially for the elderly, because the adaptability and functional reserves of the geriatric patients are more limited and 'therapeutic windows' tend to be open for a shorter period. Functional consequences and mortality rapidly elevates with the length of the delay, e.g., initiating any treatment (pneumonia, etc.).

The clinical picture of the disease in multi-morbid elderly persons is often represented by non-specific and universal symptoms [38]. Response of the brain in advanced age is typically characterized by stereotypical neurological and psychiatric signs caused by encephalopathy from the secondary decompensation of the brain activity. The cerebrum is generally the most sensitive and frail organ among all in decreasing activity in geriatric patients. Less resistant involutional brain is easily prone to decompensation by hypoperfusion, hypoxemia, impaired microcirculation, systemic inflammatory response, the influence of drugs or their discontinuation, ion imbalance, hypoglycemia or other extracranial influences.

POLYPHARMACY: WHAT IT MEANS IN CLINICAL PRACTICE?

The target of this chapter is presenting a practically orientated syndrome called generally polypharmacy from the geriatrician's viewpoint. The elderly population is extremely heterogeneous group of old people not only from the medical viewpoint (disability, different morbidity and limited mobility etc.) but also social problems, dependency on other persons help, loneliness etc.) [27, 77]. The therapeutic range ('window') gets narrow, compliance decreases, interindividual variability of the efficiency increases and the risk of drug interactions and side effects of medication increases as well [82].

Typical phenomenon accompanying elderly people (especially 75 y. or older) is multi-morbidity which is often in various combinations together with geriatric syndromes [50, 80].

Polypharmacy [16, 51] usually defined as ≥ 5 drugs or sometimes also *excessive polypharmacy* as medication, e.g., ≥ 10 different medications (especially in the 'oldest old' group, e.g., ≥ 85 y. old) [41, 87].

The higher age-related multi-morbidity as mentioned above as it is closely linked to drug therapy of diseases in advanced age [97]. A growing number of seniors and still relatively little attention paid to this fact in the broader medical community makes this issue clinically very important in a practical view. According to Gómez's results [42] polypharmacy is associated with increased risk of mortality in elderly people. These dates underline the need for greater attention and deeper knowledge of at least the basics of geronto-pharmacology and its specifics in the wider medical community - including not only knowledge of changes in pharmacodynamics and pharmacokinetics in the elderly, but also drug interactions, adverse drug reactions and potentionally inappropriate medication in the elderly.

The doctor, nowadays, thanks to a very wide variety of drugs and advances in technology dosage forms can select medicine almost 'tailor-made' for each patient [114]. This option, however, on the other hand, brings some difficulties. Because of this, even serious diseases can be difficult to detect and proceed subclinically. First of all it is very demanding on the doctor´s expertise and their orientation in available medicines and detailed knowledge of their opportunities and potential risks [65]. For physicians in clinical practice there are sometimes problems with availability of recent studies´ results. The therapeutic efforts may initially lead to an entirely justified and effective drug therapy which can easily change into polypharmacy with potential health risks to the patient, despite declining compliance and the increasing costs of therapy [57].

The current demographic situation determines the contemporary global trend of increasing absolute and relative numbers of older people [20, 21, 120]. This is most noticeable among people of very old and disabled old persons requiring complicated professional care [14, 80, 87]. In the process of selecting the optimal medication for the elderly there must always be taken into account dose regimens of drugs and drug interaction [39].

Although both expressions: polypharmacy and polypragmasia are close to each other lexically and sometimes are mixed up by a professional public, they cannot be declared linguistically identical. *Polypharmacy*, often justified and effective, in old age depends primarily on co-existing multi-morbidity [4, 16, 33]. Although the individual diseases are quite correctly detected and optimally treated according to EBM (evidence-based medicine), often the threats of possible pharmacological interactions recede somewhat out of our immediate attention. Due to that it can be difficult to detect serious affections. *Polypragmasia* is defined as a condition where the patient - sometimes unnecessarily and not obviously indicated - medicines used too much, too long, in excessive doses. Polypragmasia is mentioned even in the case where the patient takes just one not strictly necessary medicine. To some extent, this notion tends to show the non-coordination and the unsuitability of therapeutic procedures and measures. Polypragmasia may lead to an exponential increase in the risk of side effects and drug interactions [23].

PRESCRIBING IN THE ELDERLY: GENERALLY

People over 65 y. in industrialized countries make up 15-20% of the population [20, 120], they consume one-third of all prescription bound drugs and a nearly half of over-the-counter medicinal products (OTC) [114, 116]. Diseases are often chronic, which means that the drug, once started, is difficult, if not impossible, to abandon. The prevalence of polypharmacy in the literature a range of 5% to 78% [58], depending on the definition used the study population and the inclusion or exclusion of prescription medications. Along with the aging population and an expected doubling of the riskiest age group (85 y. and older) over the next 30 years it can also be expected that the prevalence of polypharmacy - whether measured in any way - will continue to grow [107].

Visiting a doctor is for the patient usually connected with an expectation of getting a prescription of any drug unless the prescription is right the main reason. Leaving the patient without prescription can thus sometimes lead to a patient´s feeling of being even cheated on. In addition, taking a pill for him/her is easier than losing weight, exercising and quitting smoking. This further increases the importance of properly collected drug history with respect to OTC products that we sometimes tend to underestimate [22, 86].

In prescribing we must distinguish 3 basic characteristics: 1) Overprescribing; 2) Underprescribing and 3) Inappropriate prescribing.

Overprescribing, i.e., excessive prescribing and usage of drugs [72, 89]. The exact definition of overusage of drugs and medicines does not exist. It may take of too many products at the same time or longer than it is necessary, or the dose is exceeded and not medically approved. With a large part of chronic multi-morbid patients we simply cannot do without several drugs at the same time quite often [2]. Doctors often are led to that, among others, by recommended treatment procedures when their rigid compliance can lead to substantial polypharmacy [36]. Physician in such situations will always have to rely on 'common sense' and in the context of drug history consider whether all the medicines used by the patient really are necessary.

Underprescribing, i.e., a treatment with a low dose of a medicinal product (under-dosage) or a product which could be a benefit for the patient is not prescribed at al., [9].

Inappropriate prescribing, i.e., the elderly is administered a potentially inconvenient medication [98]. Most frequently it is the risk of serious side effects or drug interactions or interactions of the drug and the illness proper [52, 91]. These are usually drugs that are commonly given to younger and middle age people without the risk of major complications and are well-tolerated [17]. These reasons have led to the fact that in the 90 years of the 20th century in the US there were formulated Beers criteria [5, 7, 28], then a list of drugs the risk in old age supplemented and amended (1991, 1997, 2003, 2012); later modified by Fick [30, 31] and McLeod [75] and now updated American Geriatric Society/ Expert Panel [1, 28].

- Drugs that should not be administered at all in the elderly patients - for example, an older type of antihypertensive drug - agonist central alpha2-adrenergic receptors - clonidine, methyldopa, or barbiturates.
- Drugs suitable only under certain conditions and in specific situations - intolerance of safer preparation. (e.g., nitrofurantoin), if the patient does not tolerate alternative chemotherapeutics.
- Drugs that although they have their reasons, but usually they are incorrectly prescribed - for example, older antidepressants in neuropathic pain.

SPECIFICS OF PHARMACOTHERAPY IN OLD AGE: COMMON CHANGES

The specifics of pharmacotherapy in old age can be characterized as follows:

- altered response to drugs due to changes in pharmacodynamics and pharmacokinetics
- increase in side effects of drugs generally higher as compared with non-old people
- elevated non-compliance in seniors
- higher incidence of drug-drug and drug-disease interactions.

Emphasis must be placed on a consistently individualized approach respecting a number of specific and complicating factors mentioned in the preceding paragraphs. The aging and old organism usually reacts differently to commonly used drugs [110]. Prevalence of drug reactions and side effects of medication elevates practically hand in hand with increasing age of the treated seniors. An older outpatient uses 4-6 drugs on average, whereas the hospitalized one uses 5-8 medicines [92]. The elderly patients living in institutional facilities consume three times more drugs as compared to the same number of individuals across the population and women twice as many as compared to men [40].

The basic requirement for pharmacotherapy in old age is simplicity, effectiveness and efficiency. In geriatric medicine symptomatic treatment widely prevails the causal one. Its side effects can significantly alter the clinical picture of diseases. Differences between the responses to the same dose in the elderly may be in the range of 4 to 40multiple of the average [9]. This wide variation in the age effect is almost the rule and it is not reflected even by the manufacturers' recommendations. Generally, the recommended dosage in so many elderly patients may be too high. The general rule is: Start with small doses and increase them slowly until a response is achieved. Wait with the increase for a period of at least three biological half-lives. The balanced level of drug is achieved after 4-5 biological half-lives are over. This is a consequence of the general laws of pharmacokinetics. It is important in geriatric pharmacotherapy to monitor the occurrence of adverse drug reactions actively and to use simple dosing regimens.

What remains problematic in geriatric prescribing is the implementation of the results of randomized clinical trials (RCT) [56, 65, 122], and rational prescribing on the evidence based medicine (EBM) [18, 68]. On one hand, seniors are not administered drugs that have proved to be effective and fully indicated with the given diagnosis and on the other they conversely sometimes take unnecessary medications with unproven or questionable efficacy or even inappropriate drugs for the elderly. Improving knowledge of senior medical education (OTC!) may in the future play a crucial role both for patients (efficiency) and for society (economically). Almost 60% of older patients do not use medications as recommended by their doctor [108].

Questions that the prescribing doctor should always ask:

- Which drug with respect to multiple morbidity and predictable drug interaction is the most suitable one?
- What is the optimal dosage?
- Is the indication of pharmaceuticals clear and unquestionable?

As mentioned above, while the majority of younger and middle-aged patients benefit with the commonly used methods of treatment, in the elderly (especially late) they are not entirely without risk. The results of large clinical studies may underestimate the risk of usage of many drugs in current clinical practice.

COMPLIANCE VS NON-COMPLIANCE

Compliance (CIE) in the elderly is the ability of the old man to understand, respect, adhere to and implement properly the doctor's instructions [107]. In geriatrics we can distinguish non-pharmacological (diet and regime measures) compliance; pharmacological one which can already be characterized as a level of compliance with a prescribed drug regimen by the patient; outpatient compliance; institutional and social compliances [83, 85].

In the pharmacological field CIE significantly decreases with the number of used drugs and a decline in self-sufficiency (impaired mobility and manual dexterity, mental deterioration, sight and hearing deficit) [2]. Compliance in the social sphere is determined by the senior loneliness, social ostracism and poverty. It is generally influenced by the character typology of the patient, type of disease, access to doctors and the nature of the treatment [19]. With concomitant use of five drugs only 1/3 to 1/2 of the elderly fully cooperate; with the combination of 10 drugs only 1/10 to 1/5 of seniors do.

Consequences of the reduced compliance are associated with a worse outcome in a relatively wide range of different diseases (diabetes, hypertension, hypercholesterolemia, coronary heart disease [33, 82]. In practice, the non-compliance situation is considered to happen, if the deviation from full compliance is up to 20-30%. A less common form of non-compliance is a situation where the patient takes too many drugs at higher doses than there was recommended.

Non-compliance is partial or up to entire inability to meet the requirements of the old man's purposeful and comprehensive treatment. It can be, according to various studies, 10-99% (with respect to increasing age, somatic diseases, any cognitive deficit, dependence and social isolation) [69, 107]. Most often, non-compliance is conditioned by omitting the drug (up to 1/2); changing dosages, time intervals and use (up to 1/4); early termination of pharmacotherapy (the patient finds side effects himself), additional usage of medication (up to 1/5) and usage in bad indication. Non-compliance increases significantly with the amount of drugs used with a dosing interval of more than once a day. The common phenomena in the senile age include problems with the use of drugs - especially if it is a complicated dosing schedule. The optimum dosing regimen is the simplest possible one with simple dosing intervals of 1 to 2 times a day.

The non-compliance proper may be intentional or unintentional. Less frequent in old age is the intentional non-compliance which is a deliberate non-cooperation of the patient with the treatment regimen (they stop taking the pills, modify the dosage, use other medicines on the basis of friends' recommendations). In geriatrics more common is the unintentional non-compliance [60] when the patient does not manage to implement the recommendations of treatment because of previously stated reasons (physical, mental or social). Patients complain that they get complex and sometimes vague recommendations on the use of medication. Their reduced cognitive capacity prevents them from remembering the information that is conveyed quickly and concisely by doctors, nurses or pharmacists. For doctors and nurses, it is important to think about options to increase patient's motivation to adhere to the treatment regimen [68, 78]. It may be increased by simplifying the dosing regimen, decreased number of drugs, reduced dosing frequency, selecting drugs with longer half-life or slow controlled release.

According to the WHO data a range of non-adherence of patients is huge and covers more than a half of patients across the whole age population with chronic diseases. This includes e.g., more than 66% of type 2 diabetes patients. Future efforts to reduce non-compliance should lead to creating support programs for patients that are targeted to support their medication [29, 111].

CHANGES IN PHARMACOKINETICS AND PHARMACODYNAMICS IN THE ELDERLY

With age the percentage of muscle tissue becomes reduced, particularly in people with low physical activity [45, 48]. Sarcopenia represents a loss of muscle mass, which is up to 13-24% in persons 65-70 years and 60% for seniors over 80 years [55, 81]. Cardiac output after the 30th year of life decreases by an average of 1% per year, peripheral vascular resistance increases and the volume of the liver decreases, as well as the blood flow through the liver and kidneys, the larger part of the cardiac output in the elderly as compared to the younger flows through the brain, heart and skeletal muscles [41, 88, 119].

Pharmacokinetics

Changes in the Absorption of Drugs

In seniors, the absorption is negatively affected from the gastrointestinal tract with hypoacidity of gastric juice. This can be contributed in the elderly frequently with usage of antacids, H_2-receptor blockers and proton pump inhibitors, which will also lead to the diminution of the gastric secretion. The result is a decrease in resorption of iron and weakly acidic substances (e.g., salicylates). The time of gastric emptying extends and gut motility slows down, through which the delay of the onset of drug action can be caused. Between the 40th and the 80th year splanchnic blood flow to an area decreases by 20-50%. As a result of atrophy of the mucosal surface the absorption area for passive drug delivery descends by up to one third and also the number of carriers for active transport (e.g., absorption of calcium) declines clinically significantly.

Changes in the Distribution of Drugs in the Body

With increasing age (up to 85 y.) the proportion of adipose tissue increases and the volume of body fluid both intracellular and extracellular decreases by about 15%. This way the space of distribution for hydrophilic drugs (e.g., digoxin and lithium) is reduced and their factual overdose threatens. On the contrary, with lipophilic drugs a distribution area increases with the rise of the proportion of the adipose tissue. These drugs may cumulate in the adipose tissue, thereby prolonging their biological half-life (diazepam and chlordiazepoxide).

The decrease of plasma albumin is not caused by physiological aging, but is a consequence of pathological conditions associated with malnutrition in chronic patients and the institutionalized elderly. This has an influence on the effect of those drugs which are bound to plasma proteins, such as e.g., warfarin (NSAID), digoxin, and theophylline. Its share in the free fraction in the blood rises and temporarily increases their effect, but simultaneously their biotransformation and elimination from the body is increased.

Changes in Biotransformation of Drugs

There is a less significant slowing of metabolic processes in the liver. They are mainly caused by atrophy of the liver, decreasing blood flow through the portal vein and some decrease in activity of biotransformation enzymes, especially cytochrome P450 (CYP3A4, CYP2D6, CYP2C9, etc.). Conjugation processes (acetylation, glucuronidation, sulfatation) occur fairly intact, but in old age disorders of dealkylation and hydroxylation (cytochrome CYP 450) occur. Changes to these enzymes, however, are intraindividually (and especially in old age) extremely variable. Hepatic clearance declines particularly for drugs with a strong first-pass effect (some beta-blockers, calcium channel blockers, morphine, zolpidem, antidepressants and others.). Their bioavailability can then be bigger in the elderly patients by 20-40%.

Changes in Renal Elimination of Drugs

From the 30th year of life, there is a linear decrease in the glomerular filtration rate by an average of 0.75 ml/min. per year. In 80 years it is 35 to 50% of what is the normal in young healthy humans. Continuously there is a declining number of functional glomeruli in more than 2/3 of very old individuals. Active tubular secretion and reabsorption decreases, too. Renal production of aldosterone and the ability to provide renal cell sodium retention is also reduced. The diminution of renal clearance is associated with the risky rising levels of digoxin, metformin, aminoglycosides, lithium, methotrexate and others.

Pharmacodynamics

Pharmacodynamics is considered a basis of the pharmacology, although the effect of substance depends largely on its pharmacokinetics. The effects of drugs are due primarily to the specific interactions of substances with biological systems - receptor mechanisms. The remedy acts through a receptor with which it interacts, and thereby induces a characteristic response [83]. Physiological changes and a loss of homeostatic flexibility lead to increased susceptibility to side effects of pharmaceuticals - e.g., hypotension after psychotropics and hemorrhage after anticoagulants. With growing age interindividual variability in dose needed to achieve a therapeutic effect increases generally.

The higher incidence of adverse drug reactions in the elderly may be caused by altered pharmacodynamics of drugs. An example may be a higher occurrence of orthostatic hypotension at antihypertensive therapy in the elderly [66, 82], because the function of the baroreceptors is decreased and so is the ability to compensate for excessive blood pressure decrease with tachycardia for reasons of decreased sensitivity of myocardial beta-receptors to impact of catecholamines. This may be contributed by a deterioration of the blood returning from the periphery due to venous insufficiency and cerebral hypoxia caused by atherosclerosis of the cerebral arteries. Orthostatic hypotension may be caused except for antihypertensive drugs by a number of other drugs, such as substances with a vasodilator properties (nitrates, alcohol, peripheral vasodilating agents, theophylline), neuroleptics and tricyclic antidepressants. Hypotension may be deteriorated among others by hypovolemia induced by diuretics. In advanced age the number and sensitivity of the beta2-receptors decrease mainly in peripheral blood vessels, which may lead to a decrease in the effect of beta-blockers.

Increased sensitivity of receptors for heparin and warfarin will mean a greater risk of potential bleeding complications in their use. Weakening of a specific organ with disease generally makes the body sensitive to other influences (e.g., side effects of drugs - digoxin, benzodiazepines, morphine, etc.) [59]. The effect of hypnotics, anxiolytics and other centrally active drugs may be altered by chronic hypoxia of the brain in atherosclerosis of cerebral arteries (delirium, cognitive deterioration, etc.). Medication with anticholinergic activity in older adults can cause confusion, urinary retention, slowing the passage through the gastrointestinal tract up to subileus.

ADVERSE DRUG EFFECTS

The incidence of adverse drug effects (ADE) generally increases with age, the number of diseases and the number of drugs. ADE in old age are generally 3-5 times higher than in middle age [105]. Simultaneously with the trend in consumption of medicines their risk will increase [27]. In old age, while taking less than three drugs in one year ADE will occur in 2% of patients. With more than ten medicines they occur in up to 17% of seniors. Recently, more and more frequently, to the expense of monotherapy, a combination of multiple drugs has been preferred.

This fact apart from the desired and expected beneficial effect of a decline in side effects and synergism in more places can bring a higher incidence of the adverse effects [99]. In the recent decades the number of new drugs has grown explosively, particularly in psychiatry and neurology [52]. Anxiolytics and antidepressants today belong to the most frequently prescribed drugs [96]. They are often needed also by elderly patients and they are increasingly used in internal and general medicine, in geriatrics and other non-psychiatric medical branches. Up to the half of all cases of non-compliance with antidepressants, antihypertensives and lipid-lowering drugs is caused by ADE [15, 97]. The most common manifestations of ADE in old age include [64, 66]: 1. Cardiovascular (orthostatic hypotension, arrhythmia, syncope, falls); 2. Gastrointestinal (anticholinergic effects - diarrhea, constipation, nausea, vomiting); 3. Statement by the central nervous system (depression, delirium, confusion, depression, extrapyramidal symptoms). ADE are the reason of 10-20% of seniors´ hospitalization. Inappropriate medication following Beerse criteria participates according to Gurwitz study [44] only in 7% of hospitalizations.

Out of all the adverse drug reactions almost 1/3 can be anticipated and through mere reduction of the medicament dose up to 2/3 of them can be eliminated [103]. The same way as we encounter atypical course of diseases due to changes in pharmacokinetics and pharmacodynamics in the elderly, we also find more often atypical adverse drug reactions in them, which in middle age are rare or do not occur at all (e.g., delirious state, depression, parkinsonism, falls, urinary incontinence etc.) [111]. Close connection with falls is demonstrated with long-acting benzodiazepines and combination therapy of four or more medications [64, 66]. These, in combination with other risk factors increase the risk of falls up to 28 times, themselves 2.5 times. Risk molecules in geriatric therapy are those which have a high interaction potential, narrow therapeutic window and the tendency to the cumulation in elimination disorders.

Faulty diagnosis of these adverse events of pharmacological treatment can mistakenly lead to administration and prescribing other drugs, the so-called "Prescribing cascade." A comprehensive assessment of medication (both prescription bound drugs and OTC) lies in their correct indication, the right dosage, and the form appropriate to intellectual abilities and somatic skills of the patient, elimination of predictable side effects and drug interactions, minimization of their impact on the patient, considering needs of an optimal time of administration of the drug - if long-term up to permanent usage - consistent monitoring of adverse events and ongoing evaluation of compliance [111].

DRUG INTERACTIONS

Interaction of drugs in the body can arise conditions that can change both quantitative and qualitative biological response of the organism as a whole [15, 52]. In clinical practice they belong to the drug risks and may be a negative consequence of the combined treatment [41]. The number of potential drug interactions grows exponentially with the number of drugs administered [71]. They can happen both in the pharmacokinetic and pharmacodynamic areas. Some drug can interact with some food (absorption, biotransformation) and herbs (St. John's Wort et al.). The clinical correlate of the risky drug interactions may be hypoglycemia, bleeding, cardiac dysrhythmia, centrally conditioned convulsions and conditions associated with changes in blood pressure (oral antiadiabetic agents, antiarrhythmics, anticoagulants, psychotropics, anticonvulsants etc.). Budnitz [15] says that improved management of antithrombotic and antidiabetic drug has the potential to reduce hospitalizations for adverse drug events in older adults.

In old age, authors indicate that ½ patients aged 57-85 y. use ≥ 5 drugs [29]. With increasing age number of drugs grows. At the same time ½ of them form an inappropriate prescribing combination (drug-drug) and 1 in 20 has a combination of drugs with a high risk. When using five drugs the probability of drug-drug interactions is 50%, when taking more than 8 medications it is almost 90%.

About the potential drug interactions there exists a huge amount of information, while only a part of them has some clinical importance. Considering the extent of the problems the best helpers are computer programs that can warn of it and offer sufficient technical information. The question in everyday clinical practice is usually how to reduce the number of drugs in a rational pharmacotherapy? It is not probably possible just to omit the least important product. Problems occur when we deal with type-2 diabetes with contemporary incidence of hypertension and dyslipidemia, possibly also coronary heart disease [65]. Doctors are aware of possible therapeutic errors. Efforts to solve this problem led to preparations which are a combination of different drugs (antihypertensives, diuretics, antidiabetic drugs, lipid-lowering medicines etc.) into a single tablet.

Reduction of excessive polypharmacy at the same time can bring a benefit for the patient's health, improve their treatment adherence and reduce the cost of drugs. Scott [97] explicitly says that no study has shown that the change (reduction) in polypharmacy decreased morbidity or mortality in seniors, but led to a decline of the ADE (35%), cost reductions and improved compliance with the leftover medication. Similarly depicts Garfinkel [39] in his study successful discontinuation in 81% of elderly patients. No significant adverse events or death were attributable to discontinuation and 88% of patients reported global improvement in health [39]. Any drug nonprescription should belong to the routine. Holmes [49] emphasizes definition of the objectives of health care in geriatric prescribing; individual therapeutic goals; anticipated life expectancy and survival chances; the need to start with a smaller dose and slowly increase up into the effect. The objectives of health care in general in the elderly may vary from curative to purely palliative care. Similarly, the individual therapeutic goals may vary from prevention to immediate treatment [39].

The ideal situation in geriatric prescribing [106] is represented by 1 prescriptor and 1 pharmacy. Each new prescriptor increases the probability of ADE by 29%. E-prescribing according to major studies can reduce inappropriate prescribing by 1-24%. Its possible impact on polypharmacy remains unclear.

INAPPROPRIATE MEDICATIONS IN THE ELDERLY

The concept of potentially inappropriate medications in the elderly was formulated by Beers; later on also McLeod and Fick; at the beginning of the 90th in the US and has been repeatedly updated and supplemented in 1991, 1997, 2003, 2012 (Beers, McLeod, Fick) [5, 7, 28, 30, 31, 74]. Originally, these drugs were defined as medicines whose risk for elderly patients exceeds the benefit of treatment [64]. Their use should always be avoided in the elderly, furthermore they are drugs which are suitable only in exceptional circumstances and drugs that have their indications in old age, but usually they are wrongly prescribed [17].

- Fixed administration in the elderly is considered irrational for low efficiency and increased risk of drug interactions (antihypertensives of type agonist central alpha2-adrenergic receptors - clonidine, methyldopa, or barbiturates).
- These drugs should be reserved for specific situations (intolerance or ineffectiveness of safer treatments (e.g., nitrofurantoin in the treatment of urinary tract infections is risky for contingent nephrotoxicity).
- Many of these drugs may be administered to middle-aged patients without complications but not in old age (tricyclic antidepressants - reserved only for neuropathic pain).

Currently, to the more frequently used European criteria the Irish criteria of potentially needless and necessary pharmacotherapeutic procedures belong, published by O'Mahony et al. 2006 - STOP/START criteria [37]. While the STOPP criteria [36, 75, 84] point out to about 1/3 of seniors with inadequate prescription; the START criteria in almost half of older patients indicate that some of the indicated remedies with respect to the diagnosis (systolic hypertension, atrial fibrillation with CHD, osteoporosis etc.) has not been prescribed at all.

CONCLUSION

Geriatric medicine and care for the elderly is a complex matter and has a long-term to permanent character. It utilizes, in addition to conventional pharmacotherapy, nonpharmacological intervention (diet and regimen measures) in combination with psychotherapy and measures in the social sphere. The development of effective approaches to multi-morbid seniors in the future will belong to the basic not only medical, but also society-wide priorities of increasing importance in the population, which still will continue to increase the share of seniors.

With each therapy it should be applied that to treat and cure the disease is always cheaper than neglect it and then manage its subsequent complications. To achieve the highest possible degree of adherence, including compliance, mutual cooperation between patients, doctors and nurses is required. Schemes of classical internal medicine in the case of geriatrics often fail and it is necessary to approach to the individual prescribing for seniors regarding a number of factors.

Pharmacotherapeutic treatment success depends on a multitude of factors. To avoid side effects of drugs and drug interactions when treating patients of all ages, it is necessary to carefully consider all the complex phenomena. These include health status of the patient, physiological and pathological changes due to age, mental state, a selection of suitable drugs and their mechanism of action, possible interactions simultaneously administered pharmaceuticals, suitable dosage forms, dosing regimen, and patient compliance on its own treatment. The problem remains in regular usage of freely available products, dietary supplements and drugs of plant origin, which should be taken on account in the third up to the half of older patients and which are not incorporated into their medication proper.

Finally, the chapter about pharmacotherapy in old age may be summarized as follows:

1. Improving the quality of life is a primary goal of pharmacotherapy in old age.
2. Complete cure of disease is not always possible.

3. If a drug therapy is needed, the age and multi-morbidity may cause that the expected effect will not come.

REFERENCES

[1] American Geriatrics Society Expert Panel on the Care of Older Adults with Multimorbidity. Guiding principles for the care of older adults with multimorbidity: an approach for clinicians. *J Am Geriatr Soc.* 2012; 60: 10, E1-E25.

[2] Anthierens S., Tansens A., Petrovic M. Qualitative insights into general practitioners views on polypharmacy. *BMC Fam Pract.*, 2010, 11, 65.

[3] Azad N., Molnar F., Byszewski A. Lessons learned from a multidisciplinary heart failure clinic for older women: a randomised controlled trial. *Age Ageing.* 2008; 37: 282-287.

[4] Balducci L., Goetz-Parten D., Steinman M. A. Polypharmacy and the management of the older cancer patient. *Ann Oncol.* 2013; 24 (suppl 7): vii36-vii40.

[5] Beers M. H., Ouslander J. G., Rollingher I. et al. Explicit criteria for determining inappropriate medication use in nursing home residents. *Arch Intern Med.* 1991; 151:1825-1832.

[6] Beers M. H., Thomas V. J., Jones T. V. (eds.) (2006) *The Merck Manual of Geriatrics* - 7th edition, Merck & Co, NY, 2006, electronic version.

[7] Beers M. H. Explicit criteria for determining potentially inappropriate medication use by the elderly: an update. *Arch Intern Med.* 1997; 157: 1531-1536.

[8] Blackburn J. A., Dulmus C. N. (editors): *Handbook of gerontology: evidence-based approaches to theory, practice, and policy*, Hoboken, N. J. Wiley, NY, 2007, p. 566.

[9] Blanco-Reina E., Ariza-Zafra G., Ocaña-Riola R., León-Ortíz M., Bellido-Estévez I. Optimizing elderly pharmacotherapy: polypharmacy vs. undertreatment. Are these two concepts related? *Eur J Clin Pharmacol.* 2015; 71(2):199-207.

[10] Bohannon R. W., Gorack W. Measurement of distance walked by older adults participating in subacute rehabilitation. *PM R.* 2015; 7(2):130-134.

[11] Boult C., Wieland G. D. Comprehensive primary care for older patients with multiple chronic conditions: 'Nobody rushes you through.' *JAMA.* 2010; 304: 1936-1943.

[12] Boyd C. M., Darer J., Boult C. et al. Clinical practice guidelines and quality of care for older patients with multiple comorbid diseases: implications for pay for performance. *JAMA* 2005; 294 (6): 716-724.

[13] Boyd C. M., Fortin M. Future of Multimorbidity Research:How Should Understanding of Multimorbidity Inform Health System Design? *Public Health Reviews*. 2010; 32: 451-474.

[14] Bronskill S. E., Gill S. S., Paterson J. M., Bell C. M., Anderson G. M., Rochon P. A. Exploring variation in rates of polypharmacy across long term care homes. *J Am Med Dir Assoc*. 2012; 13(3):309.e15-21.

[15] Budnitz D. S., Lovegrove M. C., Shehab N., Richards C. L. Emergency hospitalizations for adverse drug events in older Americans. *N Engl J Med*. 2011; 365(21):2002-2012.

[16] Bushardt R. L., Massey E. B., Simpson T. W., Ariail J. C., Simpson K. N. Polypharmacy: misleading, but manageable. *Clin Interv Aging*. 2008; 3(2):383-389.

[17] Cahir C., Fahey T., Teeling M. et al. Potentially inappropriate prescribing and cost outcomes for older people: a national population study. *Br J Clin Pharmacol*. 2010; 69(5): 543-552.

[18] Cassel C. H. K., Leipzig R., Cohen H. J., Larson E. B., Meier D. J. (Editors): *Geriatric medicine*: an evidence-based approach paperback softcover reprint of the original 4th ed., New York, Springer-Verlag Inc. 2013.

[19] Corrigan M. V., Pallaki M. General principles of hypertension management in the elderly. *Clin Geriatr Med*. 2009; 25(2):207-212.

[20] *Czech Health Statistics Yearbook 2013*. Praha: ÚZIS ČR, 2014.

[21] *Český statistický úřad*. [Citováno 2015-06-07]. Available at: https://www.czso.cz/csu/czso/souborne-publikace [in Czech].

[22] Delafuente J. C. Understanding and preventing drug interactions in elderly patients. *Crit Rev Oncol Hematol*. 2003; 48(2): 133-143.

[23] Doan J., Zakrzewski-Jakubiak H., Roy J., Turgeon J., Tannenbaum C. Prevalence and risk of potential cytochrome P450-mediated drug-drug interactions in older hospitalized patients with polypharmacy. *Ann Pharmacother*. 2013; 47(3):324-332.

[24] Dowdy D. W., Eid M. P., Sedrakyan A., Mendez-Tellez P. A., Pronovost P. J., Herridge M. S., Needham D. M: Quality of life in adult survivors of critical illness: a systematic review of the literature. *Intensive Care Med*. 2005; 31: 611-620.

[25] Duthie E. H., Katz P. R. and Malone M. L (eds.): *The practice of geriatrics* 4th ed., Philadelphia: Saunders Elsevier, 2007, p. 681.

[26] Emmett K. R. Nonspecific and atypical presentation of disease in the older patient. *Geriatrics* 1998; 53 (2), 50-52, 58-60.

[27] Evans D. C., Cook C. H., Christy J. M., Murphy C. V., Gerlach A. T., Eiferman D., Lindsey D. E., Whitmill M. L., Papadimos T. J., Beery P. R. 2nd, Steinberg S. M., Stawicki S. P. Comorbidity-polypharmacy scoring facilitates outcome prediction in older trauma patients. *J Am Geriatr Soc*. 2012; 60(8):1465-1470.

[28] Expert Panel. American Geriatrics Society updated Beers Criteria for potentially inappropriate medication use in older adults. American Geriatrics Society 2012 Beers Criteria Update. *J Am Geriatr Soc*. 2012; 60:616-631.

[29] Farrell B., Shamji S., Monahan A., Merkley V. F. Reducing polypharmacy in the elderly: Cases to help you "rock the boat." *CPJ/RPC*., 2013;146 (5): 243-244.

[30] Fick D. M., Cooper J. W., Wade W. E. Updating the Beers' criteria for potentially inappropriate medication use in older adults. *Arch Intern Med*. 2003; 163: 2716-2724.

[31] Fick D. M., Waller J. L., McLean Jr. et al. Potentially inappropriate medication use in a Medicare-managed care population: association with higher costs and utilization. *J Managed Care Pharm*. 2001;7: 407-413.

[32] Fortin M., Hudon C., Haggerty J. et al. Prevalence estimates of multimorbidity: a comparative study of two sources. *BMC Health Serv Res*. 2010; 10:111 http://www.biomedcentral.com/1472-6963/10/111.

[33] Franchini M., Pieroni S., Fortunato L., Molinaro S., Liebman M. Polypharmacy among the elderly: analyzing the co-morbidity of hypertension and diabetes. *Curr Pharm Des*. 2015; 21(6):791-805.

[34] Fravel M. A., McDanel D. L., Ross M. B., Moores K. G., Starry M. J. Special considerations for treatment of type 2 diabetes mellitus in the elderly. *American Journal of Health-System Pharmacy*. 2011; 68(6): 500-509.

[35] Fried L. P., Ferrucci L., Darer J., Williamson J. D., Anderson G. Untangling the concepts of disability, frailty, and comorbidity: implications for improved targeting and care. *J Gerontol A Biol Sci Med Sci*. 2004; 59 (3): 255-263.

[36] Gallagher P., O'Mahony D. STOPP (Screening Tool of Older Persons' potentially inappropriate Prescriptions): application to acutely ill elderly patients and comparison with Beers' criteria. *Age Ageing*. 2008; 37: 673-679.

[37] Gallagher P., Ryan C., Byrne S., Kennedy J., O'Mahony D. Screening
      Tool of Older Persons' potentially inappropriate Prescriptions (STOPP)
      and Screening Tool to Alert doctors to Right Treatment (START):
      Validation and application to hospitalised elderly patients. *Age Ageing*
      2008; 37: 56.
[38] Gammack J. K. and Morley J. E. (eds.): *Geriatric medicine*, Philadel-
      phia: Saunders, 2006.
[39] Garfinkel D., Mangin D. Feasibility study of a systematic approach for
      discontinuation of multiple medications in older adults: addressing
      polypharmacy. *Arch Intern Med.* 2010 Oct 11; 170(18):1648-1654.
[40] Gokce Kutsal Y., Barak A., Atalay A., Baydar T., Kucukoglu S., Tuncer
      T., Hizmetli S., Dursun N., Eyigor S., Saridogan M., Bodur H., Canturk
      F., Turhanoglu A., Arslan S., Basaran A. Polypharmacy in the elderly: a
      multicenter study. *J Am Med Dir Assoc.* 2009; 10(7):486-490.
[41] Golchin N., Frank S. H., Vince A., Isham L., Meropol S. B.
      Polypharmacy in the elderly. *J Res Pharm Pract.* 2015;4(2):85-88.
[42] Gómez C., Vega-Quiroga S., Bermejo-Pareja F., Medrano M. J., Louis
      E. D., Benito-León J. Polypharmacy in the Elderly: A Marker of
      Increased Risk of Mortality in a Population-Based Prospective Study
      (NEDICES). *Gerontology.* 2015; 61(4):301-309.
[43] Grossman S. Management of type 2 diabetes mellitus in the elderly: role
      of the pharmacist in a multidisciplinary health care team. *J Muldiscip
      Healthc*; 2011; 4: 149-154.
[44] Gurwitz J. H. Polypharmacy: a new paradigm for quality drug therapy in
      the elderly? *Arch Intern Med.* 2004, 164, 18, 1957-1959.
[45] Halter J., Ouslander J., Tinetti M. et al. (eds). *Hazzard's Geriatric
      Medicine and Gerontology*, Sixth Edition (Principles of Geriatric
      Medicine & Gerontology), 6th edition, New York: McGraw-Hill
      Professional, 2009.
[46] Hazzard W. R. Scientific progress in geriatric syndromes: earning an 'A'
      on the 2007 report card on academic geriatrics. *J Am Geriatr Soc.* 2007;
      55: 794-796.
[47] Hegyi L., Krajčík Š. a kol., *Geriatria.* Bratislava: Herba, spol. sr.o., 2010
      [in Slovac].
[48] Heiss H. W. (ed): *Altersmedizin aktuell.* Interdisziplinäre geriatrische
      Versorgung, 32. Ergänzungslieferung. Heidelberg, München, Landsberg,
      Frechen, Hamburg: Ecomed MEDIZIN, 2014 [in German].

[49] Holmes H. M., Hayley D. C., Alexander G. C., Sachs G. A. Reconsidering medication appropriateness for patients late in life. *Arch Intern Med.* 2006, 166, 6, 605-609.

[50] Hovstadius B., Astrand B., Petersson G. Assessment of regional variation in polypharmacy. *Pharmacoepidemiol Drug Saf.* 2010; 19(4): 375-83.

[51] Hovstadius B., Hovstadius K., Astrand B., Petersson G. Increasing polypharmacy - an individual-based study of the Swedish population 2005-2008. *BMC Clin Pharmacol.* 2010; 10:16.

[52] Hovstadius B., Petersson G., Hellström L., Ericson L. Trends in inappropriate drug therapy prescription in the elderly in Sweden from 2006 to 2013: assessment using national indicators. *Drugs Aging.* 2014; 31(5):379-386.

[53] Chitty K. M., Evans E., Torr J. J., Iacono T., Brodaty H., Sachdev P., Trollor J. N. Central nervous system medication use in older adults with intellectual disability: Results from the successful ageing in intellectual disability study. *Aust N Z J Psychiatry.* 2015 May 27. pii: 0004867415587951. [Epub ahead of print].

[54] Inouye S. K., Studenski S., Tinetti M. E., Kuchel G. A: Geriatric syndromes: clinical, research, and policy implications of a core geriatric concept. *J. Am. Geriatr. Soc.* 2007; 55: 780-7 91.

[55] Jacobs J. M., Maaravi Y., Cohen A. et al. Changing profile of health and function from age 70 to 85 years. *Gerontology* 2012; 58: 313-321.

[56] Jadad A. R., To M. J., Emara M., Jones J. Consideration of multiple chronic diseases in randomized controlled trials. *JAMA.* 2011; 306: 2670-2672.

[57] Jódar-Sánchez F., Malet-Larrea A., Martín J. J., García-Mochón L., López Del Amo M. P., Martínez-Martínez F., Gastelurrutia-Garralda M. A., García-Cárdenas V., Sabater-Hernández D., Sáez-Benito L., Benrimoj S. I. Cost-utility analysis of a medication review with follow-up service for older adults with polypharmacy in community pharmacies in Spain: the conSIGUE program. *Pharmacoeconomics.* 2015;33(6): 599-610.

[58] Jorgensen T., Johansson S., Kennerfalk A., Wallander M., Svardsudd K. Prescription drug use, diagnoses, and healthcare utilization among the elderly. *Ann Pharmacother.* 2001; 35(9): 1004-1009.

[59] Justiniano C. F., Coffey R. A., Evans D. C., Jones L. M., Jones C. D., Bailey J. K., Miller S. F., Stawicki S. P. Comorbidity-polypharmacy score predicts in-hospital complications and the need for discharge to

extended care facility in older burn patients. *J Burn Care Res.* 2015; 36(1):193-196.

[60] Jyrkkä J., Mursu J., Enlund H., Lönnroos E. Polypharmacy and nutritional status in elderly people. *Curr Opin Clin Nutr Metab Care.* 2012; 15(1):1-6.

[61] Kalvach Z., Zadák Z., Jirák R., Zavázalová H., Holmerová I., Weber P. *A kolektiv: Geriatrické syndromy a geriatrický pacient.* Praha: Galén, 2008 [in Czech].

[62] Keeler E., Guralnik J. M., Tian H. et al. The impact of functional status on life expectancy in older persons. *J Gerontol A Biol Sci Med* 2010; 65: 727-733.

[63] Kimball J. W. *Kimball's biology pages.* [Cited 2015-06-07]. Available from: Available from: www.users.rcn.com/jkimball.ma.ultranet/biology-pages/W/welcome/hml.

[64] Kojima T., Akishita M., Nakamura T., Nomura K., Ogawa S., Iijima K., Eto M., Ouchi Y. Polypharmacy as a risk for fall occurrence in geriatric outpatients. *Geriatr Gerontol Int.* 2012; 12(3):425-430.

[65] Koper D., Kamenski G., Flamm M., Böhmdorfer B., Sönnichsen A. Frequency of medication errors in primary care patients with polypharmacy. *Fam Pract.* 2013; 30(3):313-319.

[66] Kuschel B. M., Laflamme L., Möller J. The risk of fall injury in relation to commonly prescribed medications among older people: a Swedish case-control study. *Eur J Public Health.* 2015; 25(3):527-532.

[67] Kuschel B. M., Laflamme L., Möller J. The risk of fall injury in relation to commonly prescribed medications among older people--a Swedish case-control study. *Eur J Public Health.* 2015; 25(3):527-532.

[68] Lally F. (Editor), Roffe Ch. (Editor): *Geriatric Medicine: an evidence-based approach Paperback*, 1 edition. Oxford, London; Oxford University Press: 2014.

[69] Leendertse A. J., de Koning G. H., Goudswaard A. N., Belitser S. V., Verhoef M., de Gier H. J., Egberts A. C., van den Bemt P. M. Preventing hospital admissions by reviewing medication (PHARM) in primary care: an open controlled study in an elderly population. *J Clin Pharm Ther.* 2013; 38(5):379-387.

[70] Linnebur S. A., Vande Griend J. P., Metz K. R., Hosokawa P. W., Hirsch J. D., Libby A. M. Patient-level medication regimen complexity in older adults with depression. *Clin Ther.* 20141; 36(11):1538-1546.

[71] Longo, D., Fauci, A., Kasper, D. et al. *Harrison's Principles of Internal Medicine.* 18th ed. United States: NY; McGraw-Hill Medical Publishing Division 2011.

[72] Manias E., Kusljic S., Berry C., Brown E., Bryce E., Cliffe J., Smykowsky A. Use of the Screening Tool of Older Person's Prescriptions (STOPP) in older people admitted to an Australian hospital. *Australas J Ageing.* 2015; 34(1):15-20.

[73] Marengoni A., Angleman S., Melis R. et al. Aging with multimorbidity: a systematic review of the literature. *Ageing Res Rev.* 2011; 10: 430-439.

[74] Matějovská Kubešová H., Weber P., Meluzínová H., Matějovský J. Senioři a kardiovaskulární medikace. *Vnitř Lék*, 57, 2011, 561-570.

[75] McLeod P. J., Huang A. R., Tamblyn R. M., Gayton D. C. Defining inappropriate practices in prescribing for elderly people: a national consensus panel. *CMAJ.* 1997; 156:385-391.

[76] Menotti A., Mulder I., Nissinen A. et al. Prevalence of morbidity and multimorbidity in elderly male populations and their impact on 10-year all-cause mortality: The FINE study (Finland, Italy, Netherlands, Elderly). *J Clin Epidemiol* 2001; 54 (7): 680-686.

[77] Moen J., Antonov K., Larsson C. A. et al. Factors associated with multiple medication use in different age groups. *Ann Pharmacother.* 2009; 43(12): 1978-1985.

[78] Moody H. R. *Aging: concepts and controversies*, 5th ed., Thousand Oaks, Calif., London: Pine Forge, c2006.

[79] Moral R. R., Torres L. A., Ortega L. P., Larumbe M. C., Villalobos A. R., García J. A., Rejano J. M. Collaborative Group ATEM-AP Study. Effectiveness of motivational interviewing to improve therapeutic adherence in patients over 65 years old with chronic diseases: A cluster randomized clinical trial in primary care. *Patient Educ Couns.* 2015; 98(8):977-983.

[80] Morley J. E., Caplan G. Cesari M. International Survey of Nursing Home Research Priorities. *JAMDA.* 2014; 15(5): 309-312.

[81] Morley J. E., Vellas B., van Kan G. A., Anker S. D., Bauer J. M., Bernabei R., Cesari M., Chumlea W. C., Doehner W., Evans J., Fried L. P., Guralnik J. M., Katz P. R., Malmstrom T. K., McCarter R. J., Gutierrez Robledo L. M., Rockwood K., von Haehling S., Vandewoude M. F., Walston J. Frailty consensus: a call to action. *J Am Med Dir Assoc.* 2013; 14(6): 392-397.

[82] Nechbaa R. B., Moncif El M'barki Kadiric, Mounia Bennani-Ziatnid, Zeggwaghe A. A., Abdelhalim Mesfiouib. Difficulty in managing

polypharmacy in the elderly: Case report and review of the literature. *Journal of Clinical Gerontology and Geriatrics.* 2015;6(1):30-33.

[83] Nobil A., Licata G., Salerno F., Pasina L., Tettamanti M., Franchi C., De Vittorio L., Marengoni A., Corrao S., Iorio A., Marcucci M., Mannucci P. M., SIMI Investigators. Polypharmacy, length of hospital stay, and in-hospital mortality among elderly patients in internal medicine wards. The REPOSI study. *Eur J Clin Pharmacol.* 2011; 67(5):507-519.

[84] Núñez Montenegro A. J., Montiel Luque A., Martín Aurioles E., Torres Verdú B., Lara Moreno C., González Correa J. A., en representación del grupo Polipresact. Adherence to treatment, by active ingredient, in patients over 65 years on multiple medication. *Aten Primaria.* 2014 May; 46(5):238-245. [Article in Spanish].

[85] O'Reilly V., Hartigan I., Coleman A., Morrissey C., O'Sullivan C., O'Connor M. et al. A new Screening Tool of Older Persons Prescriptions (STOPP) in the acute hospital setting. *Irish J Med Sci* 2004; 173: 12-13.

[86] Olsson I. N., Runnamo R., Engfeldt P. Drug treatment in the elderly: an intervention in primary care to enhance prescription quality and quality of life. *Scand J Prim Health Care.* 2012; 30(1):3-9.

[87] Onder G., Liperoti R., Fialova D., Topinkova E., Tosato M., Danese P., Gallo P. F., Carpenter I., Finne-Soveri H., Gindin J., Bernabei R., Landi F., SHELTER Project. Polypharmacy in nursing home in Europe: results from the SHELTER study. *J Gerontol A Biol Sci Med Sci.* 2012;67(6): 698-704.

[88] Pathy M. S., John, Finucane P. (eds.): *Geriatric Medicine: Problems and Practice paperback*; NY: Springer, 2014.

[89] Payne R. A., Avery A. J. Polypharmacy: one of the greatest prescribing challenges in general practice. *Br J Gen Pract.* 2011 Feb; 61(583):83-84.

[90] Pirlich M., Schütz T., Norman K., Gastell S., Lübke H. J., Bischoff S. C., Bolder U., Frieling T., Güldenzoph T. H., Hahn K., Jauch K. W., Schindler K., Stein J., Volkert D., Weimann A., Werner J. J., Wolf C., Zürcher G., Bauer P., Lochs H., German hospital malnutrition study. *Clinical Nutrition* 2006; 5: 563-572.

[91] Prithviraj G. K., Koroukian S., Margevicius S., Berger N. A., Bagai R., Owusu C. Patient Characteristics Associated with Polypharmacy and Inappropriate Prescribing of Medications among Older Adults with Cancer. *J Geriatr Oncol.* 2012; 3(3):228-237.

[92] Rai Gurcharan S. and Mulley G. P. (eds.): *Elderly medicine: a training guide*, 2nd ed., Edinburgh, Churchill Livingstone Elsevier: 2007.

[93] Ramage-Morin P. *Medication use among senior Canadians*. Health Rep., 2009; 20(1):37-44.

[94] Rivera-Fernandez R., Navarrete-Navarro P., Fernandez-Mondejar E., Rodriguez-Elvira M., Guerrero-Lałpez F., Vazquez-Mata G., Project for the Epidemiological Analysis of Critical Care Patients (PAEEC) Group: Six-year mortality and quality of life in critically ill patients with chronic obstructive pulmonary disease. *Crit. Care. Med.* 2006; 34: 2317-2324.

[95] Rockwood K., Song X., MacKnight C. et al. A global clinical measure of fitness and frailty in elderly people. *CMAJ*. 2005; 173: 489-495.

[96] Salive M. E. Multimorbidity in older adults. *Epidemiol Rev.* 2013; 35: 75-83.

[97] Sare G. M., Gray L. J., Bath P. M. Association between hormone replacement therapy and subsequent arterial and venous vascular events: a meta-analysis. *Eur Heart J.* 2008; 29: 2031-2041.

[98] Scott I. A., Gray L. C., Martin J. H., Mitchell C. A. Minimizing inappropriate medications in older populations: a 10-step conceptual framework. *Am J Med.* 2012, 125, 6, 529-537.

[99] Sganga F., Landi F., Ruggiero C., Corsonello A., Vetrano D. L., Lattanzio F., Cherubini A., Bernabei R., Onder G. Polypharmacy and health outcomes among older adults discharged from hospital: results from the CRIME study. *Geriatr Gerontol Int.* 2015; 15(2):141-146.

[100] Shah B., Hajjar E. Polypharmacy, adverse drug reactions and geriatric syndromes. *Clin Geriatr Med* 2012; 28:173-186.

[101] Sharma V., Aggarwalb S., Sharma A. Diabetes in Elderly. *J Endocrinol Metab*. 2011; 1(1): 9-13.

[102] Schäfer I., Hansen H., Schön G. et al. The German MultiCare-study: Patterns of multimorbidity in primary health care - protocol of a prospective cohort study. *BMC Health Serv Res*. 2009; 11 (9): http:// www.biomedcentral.com/1472-6963/9/145.

[103] Schäfer I., von Leitner E. C., Schön G. et al. Multimorbidity patterns in the elderly: a new approach of disease clustering identifies complex interrelations between chronic conditions. *PLoS One*. 2010; 5 (12): e15941. www.plosone.org.

[104] Schuling J., Gebben H., Veehof L. J., Haaijer-Ruskamp F. M. Deprescribing medication in very elderly patients with multimorbidity: the view of Dutch GPs. A qualitative study. *BMC Fam Pract*. 2012; 13: 56.

[105] Siccama R. N., Janssen K. J., Verheijden N. A., Oudega R., Bax L., van Delden J. J., Moons K. G. Systematic review: diagnostic accuracy of

clinical decision rules for venous thromboembolism in elderly. *Ageing Res Rev.* 2011; 10: 304-313.

[106] Sinclair A. J., Paolisso G., Castro M., Bourdel-Marchasson I., Gadsby R., Rodriguez Mañas L., European Diabetes Working Party for Older People. European Diabetes Working Party for Older People 2011 clinical guidelines for type 2 diabetes mellitus. Executive summary. *Diabetes Metab.* 2011; 37(Suppl. 3): S27-S38.

[107] Steinman M. A., Handler S. M., Gurwitz J. H., Schiff G. D., Covinsky K. E. Beyond the prescription: medication monitoring and adverse drug events in older adults. *J Am Geriatr Soc.* 2011; 59: 1513-1520.

[108] Stortz J. N., Lake J. K., Cobigo V., Ouellette-Kuntz H. M., Lunsky Y. Lessons learned from our elders: how to study polypharmacy in populations with intellectual and developmental disabilities. *Intellect Dev Disabil.* 2014; 52(1):60-77.

[109] Szanton S. L., Seplaki C. L., Thorpe R. J. Jr., Allen J. K., Fried L. P. Socioeconomic status is associated with frailty: the Women's Health and Aging Studies. *J. Epidemiol. Community Health.* 2010; 64(1): 63-67.

[110] Topinková E. *Zvláštnosti farmakoterapie ve stáří* [online]. Available at: [cit. 2012-02-13]. <http://www.edukafarm.cz/clanek.php?id=548 [in Czech].

[111] Valderas J. M., Starfield B., Sibbald B. et al. Defining comorbidity: implications for understanding health and health services. *Ann Fam Med.* 2009; 7: 357-363.

[112] Van der Cammen T. J., Rajkumar C., Onder G., Sterke C. S., Petrovic M. Drug cessation in complex older adults: time for action. *Age Ageing.* 2014; 43(1):20-25.

[113] Weber P., Ambrošová P., Weberová D. et al. Geriatrické syndromy a syndrom frailty zlatý grál geriatrické medicíny. *Vnitř Lék* 2011; 57 (6), E2010_18 online.

[114] Werder S., Preskorn S. Managing polypharmacy: Walking the fine line between help and harm. *Current Psychiatry Online.* 2003 2(2). Avalaible at: www.currentpsychiatry.com/UserInputInfo.asp?AID=601&PID=0.

[115] Williams B., Chang A., Landefeld C., Ahalt C., Conant R., Chen H. (Eds.): *Current Diagnosis and Treatment*: Geriatrics 2E 2 edition.

[116] Williams C. Using medications appropriately in older adults. Am Fam McGraw-Hill Education/Medical; 2014. *Physician.* 2002; 66(10): 1917-1924.

[117] Williams M. E. *Geriatric physical diagnosis: a guide to observation and assessment*, Jefferson, N. C.: McFarland & Co., c2008.

[118] Wilson M. M. G. *Liver and gall bladder*. In: Pathy M. S. John, Sinclair Alan J., Morley John E. (eds.): Principles and practice of geriatric medicine, 4th ed., Chichester: Wiley, 2006.

[119] Woodford, H., *Essential geriatrics*, Abingdon: Radcliffe, 2007.

[120] Wrobel N. Demografieinduzierte Multi-Morbidität - Komplexleistung Im DRG-Vergütungssystem. *Recht und Politik im Gesundheitswesen* 2008; 14 (1): 7-10.

[121] Zulman D. M., Sussman J. B., Chen X., Cigolle C. T., Blaum C. S., Hayward R. A. Examining the evidence: a systematic review of the inclusion and analysis of older adults in randomized controlled trials. *J Gen Intern Med*. 2011; 26: 783-790.

INDEX

aldehydes, 75
aldosterone, 124
alertness, 16
alkalosis, 88
allele, 104
ALT, 27
alters, 68, 71, 72, 84
amines, 4
amino, 7, 38, 57, 67, 70, 73, 82, 83, 87
amino acid(s), 38, 67, 70, 73, 82, 83, 87
aminoglycosides, 124
amnesia, 30
analgesic, 16, 19, 25, 26, 41
anaphylaxis, 29
angina, 94, 113
angioedema, 29
anorexia, 111
anoxia, 84
ANS, 102
antacids, 122
antagonism, 80
anterograde amnesia, 32
anticholinergic, 3, 4, 125
anticholinergic effect, 125
anticholinergic properties, 3, 4
anticonvulsant(s), vii, 1, 2, 4, 27, 32, 44, 71, 99, 127
antidepressant(s), vii, 1, 2, 3, 10, 13, 35, 119, 123, 124, 125, 128
antihypertensive drugs, 124
antioxidant, ix, 49, 52, 53, 55, 56, 58, 60, 63, 69, 70, 76, 77, 78, 80, 83
antioxidant enzymes, ix, 49, 52, 77, 83
antipsychotic(s), vii, 1, 3, 31, 100
antipyretic, 25
anxiety, 10, 16, 21, 30, 50, 58, 77, 79, 87, 91, 99, 101
anxiety disorder, 10, 30
anxiolytics, vii, 1, 2, 3, 125
anxiousness, 100
APAP, viii, 16, 18, 25, 26, 27, 28, 29, 37
apoptosis, 66, 74, 75, 77, 78, 79, 82, 83
arginine, 54, 64, 74
arrest, 35
arrhythmia, 3, 125

aspartate, 27, 50, 57, 73, 77, 78, 80, 87
asphyxia, 80
aspiration, 36, 95, 103
aspiration pneumonia, 36
assessment, x, 35, 46, 84, 90, 91, 96, 98, 99, 101, 102, 105, 108, 126, 134, 139
asthma, 94
ataxia, 3, 35, 99
atherosclerosis, 110, 113, 124, 125
ATLAS, 42
atoms, 52
ATP, 52, 58, 60, 62, 79, 83
atrial fibrillation, 129
atrophy, 53, 123
autonomy, 110
autopsy, 2, 3, 4, 5, 6, 9, 10, 11, 13

B

bacteria, 12
barbiturates, 2, 13, 36, 119, 128
base, 55, 94, 104
beneficial effect, 125
benefits, 19
benign, 28
benzodiazepine(s), viii, 2, 8, 12, 13, 16, 30, 45, 46, 74, 75, 79, 95, 96, 97, 98, 99, 125, 126
beta blocker, 96, 99, 100
beverages, 7
bile, 26
bioavailability, 20, 35, 75, 123
biochemistry, 72
bioconversion, 6
biological systems, 124
biosynthesis, 55
bleeding, 125, 126
blood, vii, xi, 2, 5, 6, 7, 9, 12, 13, 16, 23, 35, 36, 54, 78, 88, 90, 99, 102, 109, 122, 123, 124, 126
blood flow, xi, 109, 122, 123
blood pressure, 16, 36, 99, 124, 127
boat, 132
body composition, 115
body fat, 115

evidence, ix, xi, 4, 19, 36, 42, 44, 49, 54, 61,
67, 71, 78, 98, 99, 104, 108, 117, 120,
130, 131, 135, 140
examinations, viii, 2
excitability, 32
excitation, 87
excitatory postsynaptic potentials, 58
excitotoxicity, 57, 61, 65, 67, 70, 71, 81, 82
exclusion, 118
exercise(s), 46, 115
expertise, xi, 109, 117
exposure, 16, 23, 26, 31, 33, 43, 53, 55, 59,
61, 72

F

failure to thrive, 111
false negative, 35
false positive, 35
family support, 24
fat, 97, 111, 115
fatal arrhythmia, 3
fever, 94
fibers, 77
fibroblasts, 61
filtration, 124
Finland, 136
fitness, 138
flexibility, 124
fluid, 53, 94, 95
fluid balance, 94, 95
Flumazenil, viii, 16, 36, 37, 47
folic acid, 72
food, 126
Food and Drug Administration (FDA), 20,
36
force, 51, 60
Ford, 39
formation, 5, 7, 43, 54, 67
frailty, 110, 111, 132, 136, 138, 139
free radicals, 64, 82
fructose, 80

G

GABA, viii, 3, 4, 16, 18, 32, 36, 50, 51, 74,
86, 87, 96, 97, 99, 100, 101, 103
gait, 111
gait disorders, 111
gas chromatography (GC), 5
gas chromatography mass spectrometry
(GC/MS), 5
gastrectomy, 13
gastric mucosa, 82
gastrointestinal tract, xi, 4, 36, 109, 122,
125
gel, 30
gene expression, 66, 70
general practitioner, 130
generalized tonic-clonic seizure, 87
genes, 56, 67, 70, 76
genetic disease, 56
genetic predisposition, 87
genetics, 87
geriatric syndromes, 110, 111, 133, 138
gerontology, 130
glucose, 95, 114
glucose tolerance, 114
glutamate, ix, 49, 50, 55, 56, 57, 58, 59, 61,
63, 65, 66, 67, 68, 69, 70, 71, 72, 73, 74,
77, 79, 80, 81, 82, 83, 84, 87
glutamine, 65, 82
glutathione, 26, 27, 28, 43, 44, 55, 56, 71
glycine, 103
granules, 4
growth, 66, 111, 113, 115
guanine, 55
guidelines, xi, 108, 131, 139

H

half-life, 20, 21, 22, 27, 37, 38, 100, 122,
123
hallucinations, 19, 35, 87, 88, 91, 100, 101,
102, 104
head injury, 95
head trauma, 103

I

protein carbonyl, 54, 55, 62
protein kinases, 66, 72, 80
protein oxidation, ix, 49, 54, 55, 61, 64, 69,
    70, 71, 79
proteins, 26, 54, 61, 62, 66, 70, 78, 82, 84
proton pump inhibitors, 122
protons, 60
pruritus, 29
psychiatric diagnosis, 50
psychiatry, 125
psychosis, 9, 92
psychotherapy, 129
psychotropic drugs, vii, 1, 2, 4, 7, 9, 11, 13
psychotropic medications, 8
public health, 2, 23
pulmonary edema, viii, 2, 21
pumps, 61

Q

QRS complex, 3, 4
QT interval, 3, 4
quality of life, x, 108, 129, 137, 138
quantification, 5
quinone, 43

R

radicals, 52, 53, 55, 73, 80
rash, 29
reactions, xi, xii, 29, 32, 53, 70, 109, 126
Reactive Nitrogen Species, 64
reactive oxygen, ix, 49, 76, 82, 83
reactive oxygen species, ix, 49, 76, 82, 83
receptor(s), viii, ix, 2, 16, 18, 19, 20, 21, 32,
    33, 36, 39, 40, 49, 50, 51, 57, 58, 59, 63,
    65, 66, 68, 72, 74, 77, 78, 79, 80, 81, 82,
    83, 84, 86, 87, 96, 99, 100, 101, 103,
    119, 122, 124, 125, 128
recognition, 28, 29
recommendations, xi, 108, 120, 121
recovery, 103
redistribution, 5, 6, 12
rehabilitation, 19, 130

relapses, 97, 99
relatives, 113
relaxation, 30
relevance, 71, 81
repair, 56
requirement(s), 72, 76, 84, 93, 119, 121
reserves, 111, 115
residue(s), 12, 54, 67, 70
resistance, 122
resolution, 27
respiration, 19, 39
respiratory rate, 19, 22
response, 7, 16, 19, 21, 36, 39, 61, 72, 75,
    81, 98, 116, 119, 120, 124, 126
restrictions, 112
rhinorrhea, 21, 29
risk assessment, 75
risk factors, 27, 39, 78, 102, 126
rodents, 54
roots, 82
routes, viii, 15, 24, 38, 98
rules, 139

S

safety, 41
salicylates, 122
saliva, 35
sarcopenia, 111
saturation, 22
schizophrenia, 71, 75
science, 47
screening test., 5
secretion, 114, 122, 124
sedative(s), viii, 2, 9, 16, 18, 25, 31, 35, 36,
    45, 76, 87, 89, 94, 95, 97, 99
sedative medication, viii, 16
segregation, 110
seizure, viii, 4, 30, 36, 37, 49, 58, 59, 79,
    82, 95, 100, 102
selective serotonin reuptake inhibitor(s)
    (SSRI), 2, 10, 35
self-sufficiency, 110, 112, 113, 121
senescence, 110
senses, 101

T

U

V

W